DATE			
OC 26 '84			
FE 15 '85			
AP 19 '85			

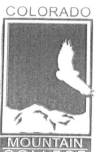

Caring for LIVESTOCK

A VETERINARY HANDBOOK

Jaime Isaac Reibel

ARCO PUBLISHING, INC.
NEW YORK

This animal husbandry guide has been written for use as a resource to complement the assistance offered by your veterinarian. It is not intended to replace the vet but rather to enable the reader to make more educated and timely use of his or her aid. The information contained in this book is for educational purposes and is not intended to replace the advice of qualified medical professionals. A veterinarian should be consulted regarding any specific medical condition. The author and publisher are not responsible for any adverse consequences resulting from the use of medications or procedures mentioned in this book.

Line drawings by Edwin Cevallos Galarza

Published by Arco Publishing, Inc.
215 Park Avenue South, New York, N.Y. 10003

Library of Congress Cataloging in Publication Data

Reibel, Jaime Isaac.
  Caring for livestock.

  Includes index.
  1. Veterinary medicine—Handbooks, manuals, etc.
I. Title.
SF751.R37 1984   616.089   83-21349
ISBN 0-668-05576-6 (Cloth Edition)

Printed in the United States of America

10 9 8 7 6 5 4 3 2 1

CONTENTS

List of Tables

ACKNOWLEDGMENTS

This book would not have made its way into print were it not for the support and assistance of numerous friends both in Ecuador and in the United States. Among those most deserving of praise are Dr. Fausto Maldonado Paredes, presently of AID, who strongly backed the idea for this guide when we worked together at PREDESUR in 1978 and 1979; Edwin "Pucho" Cevallos Galarza, the artist of this book who endured my innumerable revisions with good humor; Dr. Leonard Bull, head of the Animal Science Department, and Dr. Bill Kelly, Associate Dean of Agriculture, both of the University of Vermont.

I have been very lucky to have Madelyn Larsen as my editor. She has been constantly enthusiastic and fun to work with all the way through the project. Often we corresponded and talked from great distances, which must have been disconcerting when trying to juggle schedules and deadlines, but if so she never let on. Peter Sherred, my publisher, had the calm assurance that this animal guide was needed and continued to boost it and my spirits during the time it took to complete.

The librarians of the Facultad de Veterinaria de la Universidad Central de Quito and those of the University of Vermont in Burlington were most helpful with research and reference materials.

Thanks go to my sister and brother-in-law, Sylvia and Peter Tousley, for providing a warm haven to finish the last part of the book in. And finally, to my wife, Clara Maria, for the typing of the manuscript, all your patience, and the sharing of my work, *te adoro*.

FOREWORD

Anyone with experience in agricultural education, either vocational agriculture at the high-school level or 2- and 4-year degree programs, knows how difficult it is to find appropriate textbooks and reference books. This is especially true in the area of animal health where there is a proliferation of books at either end of the informational spectrum, but very few somewhere in the middle. There are many highly technical books appropriate for upper-level degree programs that are incomprehensible to the average producer. There are also many books available for the true beginner in animal husbandry, but they are entirely inadequate for the serious producer.

The author's goal is to provide a middle ground between the technical veterinary guides and the "back to the land" type guides, and to produce an introductory textbook for beginning students in degree programs. He remembers his own experience as a student at the University of Vermont where he formed the opinion that a solid, basic overview should precede a journey into the more technical aspects. Jaime Reibel's goals and experiences are followed and incorporated as he explains and develops each section of the book.

This book is educational and goes beyond simply conveying information. The author always proceeds from an understandable description and explanation of the particular problem to equally clear and understandable directions on how to prevent or solve the problem. It is not easy to present clear, concise explanations of technical and scientific terms, but Jaime Reibel has successfully achieved this objective.

This clarity of presentation is illustrated in the very first chapter entitled, Disease: What Is It? A clear, adequate definition of disease is presented in two paragraphs, followed by equally concise and understandable descriptions of disease transmission, how the animal fights disease, immunity, and acquired immunity. It is very easy for a writer to get involved in a lengthy, unwieldy discussion when trying to define these terms, but Jaime Reibel's treatment of this subject sets the tone for the remainder of the book. This handbook is not short on technical information or sufficient detail, but the readable and easily comprehended style sets it apart from other, similar books.

This handbook will also be an excellent reference for professionals and paraprofessionals working in developing countries. Many of the small landowners in these countries are illiterate or semiliterate and therefore unable to consume the information directly from the text, but with appropriate translation, extension-type workers and others will find Reibel's work extremely useful. The prevention and treatment of animal diseases in developing countries is a major problem and it will be a long time before there are sufficient numbers of adequately trained veterinarians and other health professionals to address the problems. The only immediate solution is to put adequate "tools" in the hands of various agriculturists, and this handbook certainly qualifies as one of these aids. It is an accurate, readable reference for agricultural workers who must provide paraprofessional animal health care.

While no text or reference book can completely satisfy every conceivable audience, this handbook does an excellent job of meeting wide-ranging needs. For those potential readers with some prior knowledge of health care it can serve as a very useful, up-to-date reference book. For those readers with no background or knowledge in health care, it can function as a basic textbook and a primary reference. In the hands of livestock producers, especially beginners and less-experienced farmers, the book will probably become worn and "dog-eared" very quickly from frequent use, often under conditions of stress.

As an agricultural educator with thirty years of experience, it is especially gratifying to see one of our graduates produce such a useful and well-written book. I hope that Jaime will be able to follow up on this very successful effort with a second book emphasizing various aspects of livestock management.

William H. Kelly
Associate Dean for Instruction
College of Agriculture
University of Vermont

1

DISEASE: WHAT IS IT?

The word *disease* literally means "not at ease." It occurs when an animal's body changes from its normal healthy condition for any number of reasons. Usually it's possible to recognize that an animal is diseased by the physical signs, or symptoms, that it shows. The various causes of disease include bacteria, viruses, protozoa, internal or external parasites, poisons, poor nutrition, injuries, and environmental factors.

All living matter is a collection of cells, the basic units that enable an animal or human being to function. Cells that do the same kind of work are grouped into tissues, and they in turn work together to ensure that the body functions properly. When this happens the animal is in good health. However, whenever cells are killed in sufficiently large numbers, or their work is disrupted the animal becomes sick and is considered diseased.

Means of Transmission

Cells are attacked by tiny pathogenic (disease causing) organisms, so small that you can't see them without using a microscope. These harmful organisms are transmitted through sexual contact, carried by external parasites such as fleas, passed through contact with objects such as carrying cases and harnesses, contact with other animals' excretions or secretions; and are carried in food, water, and air, as in the case of dust, spores, and tiny droplets.

Pathogenic microbes (another word for *microorganisms*) enter the body through breaks in the skin, as with bites and wounds, and through the nostrils, mouth and throat, ears, anus, penis, and vagina. At the same time they may already be within the body and begin to attack the cells due to some other external problem. A good example of this is the microorganisms that cause mastitis, an inflammation of the udder frequently seen in dairy cattle, but also in sows, goats, and sheep. These microorganisms are commonly found in the cow's body and may begin to attack the udder tissue because of external injury to it or as a result of insufficient milking.

How the Body Fights Harmful Microbes

Once disease-causing microbes have entered the body they begin to attack the body cells and fluids. They break them down and use them for the food and energy that they need to maintain their own bodies. As they do this, pathogenic microbes create poisons called toxins.

This process causes an inflammation in the part of the body that has been attacked. The body reacts to its injury by increasing the flow of blood to the affected part in order to remove damaged tissues. The increased blood flow raises the animal's body temperature, which decreases the release of toxins by the pathogenic microbes.

The body also fights the harmful microorganisms with phagocytes, a type of white blood cell, and with antibodies, proteins found in the blood. Antibodies either kill attacking microbes outright or neutralize them so phagocytes can finish them off. Phagocytes also make antitoxins, proteins that counteract the active properties of specific toxins, causing them to become ineffective.

Cells make specific antibodies in response to toxins, enzymes (substances that either start or speed up chemical reactions), and other chemicals. These three substances are called *antigens*. Antigens cause a restricted response: one that causes antibody production against a particular disease will not cause antibody production against any other disease. Proteins are the most antigenic substances (cause the best antibody production), followed by complex carbohydrates known as polysaccharides.

In all diseases antibodies are produced in response to specific antigens; as they neutralize them the animal becomes better. However, in some diseases, after the animal becomes well again and throughout the rest of its life, the same antibodies continue to be produced. What this means is that the animal is now protected all the time and is considered immune to that particular disease (not affected by it).

Immunity

Immunity, the power to resist a specific disease, can be natural to the species or the individual and can also be acquired. Natural species immunity means that certain diseases attack only one species. Individual immunity leaves individual animals immune to given diseases which attack others within the same species. Acquired immunity is caused by vaccines, or it occurs naturally when an animal produces its own antibodies against a disease from which it has recovered.

Natural Species Immunity

Natural species immunity leaves many species free of certain diseases that can attack only one kind of animal. The unaffected species, therefore, have no need to form antibodies against many diseases because they could never be attacked by them. For example, bovine trichomoniasis, a venereal disease in cattle that usually causes infertility or abortion in the cow, can only be contracted by cows and bulls, pigs can't get it. Likewise, hog cholera, a particularly lethal disease that affects pigs of all ages, cannot be contracted by a cow or bull.

Individual Immunity

Within a herd, flock, or group of the same species of animal there is often a variation in individual immunity to a specific disease. Newcastle disease, a virus that attacks chickens, usually kills baby chicks less than 3 weeks old. But whenever a flock has the disease some chicks less than 3 weeks old don't get sick at all; others become ill and then recover.

This individual reaction within a species to the same disease is probably caused by genetic inheritance, the collection of traits received by an animal from its parents and ancestors. Since no two animals have exactly the same traits, their natural immunities will be different in the same way that cows have different colored markings, one sow may have more teats than another, and dogs may have long or short hair.

It's important for the farmer to select animals that show immunity or resistance to disease when it comes time to breed. In this way genetic inheritance can be used to his or her advantage. Take the case of two cows equal in all aspects except that one always has mastitis (which limits its milk production), while the other one never has the disease. The farmer wants to keep a heifer from one of them. The obvious choice is the offspring of the cow that never has mastitis.

There is also a variation in individual immunity in the same species depending on the animal's age. The majority of infections attack very young and old animals most severely. One of the most important ways that young animals acquire passive resistance to disease is to drink colostrum (the first milk produced by the mother that the baby animal drinks almost immediately after it's born). Colostrum provides the baby animal with the vitamins, minerals, and maternal antibodies it needs to protect it from infection in the first few weeks of its life. Baby birds receive the maternal antibodies they need from the yolk of the egg from which they develop.

Acquired Immunity

There are two kinds of acquired immunity, active and passive. Active immunity occurs when an animal produces its own antibodies after having survived an attack of a particular disease. The disease can be contracted either naturally or artificially. By artificially, we mean when the animal is injected with vaccines, bacterins, or toxins produced by the infection. Intentionally injecting an animal with any one of these three solutions in order to cause an actively acquired immunity is called vaccination.

Vaccines are preparations of living, but weakened or diluted viruses, that are injected into an animal's body to intentionally infect it with a mild form of disease. This stimulates the cells and connective tissue to produce antibodies, also called immune bodies, which then fight the infection.

Bacterins are suspensions of killed disease-causing bacteria placed in either a salt solution (equal to the strength of the one found in body fluids) or in oil. They also cause cells to produce antibodies.

Passive immunity is produced in one animal by injecting it with immune blood serum taken from another animal. The immune bodies (antibodies) produced in the actively immune animal are the component in the immune blood serum that gives passive immunity to the other animal. There are two kinds of immune bodies that can be produced. Those that work on bacteria are called antibacterial, for example, antianthrax serum. (See section on "Anthrax," p. 170, in Chapter 16, General Diseases of Domestic Animals.) Those that act on toxins are called *antitoxins*; an example is tetanus antitoxin. (See section on "Tetanus," p. 187, also in Chapter 16.)

Serum is produced in the following manner: when red and white blood cells are removed from an animal's blood, the remaining fluid is called *plasma*. Plasma is made of fibrinogen, a protein that makes blood clot, and serum, the clear to yellowish liquid that separates from a blood clot when it begins to harden and shrink. Take out the fibrinogen and only the serum is left.

Only healthy animals are used to produce immune blood serum—usually horses, because it is possible to remove large quantities of blood from them without harm.

In order to produce antitoxin, the horse is injected with a small amount of a specific toxin; to make antibacterial serum the animal is injected with specific disease-causing bacteria. The antibodies are produced, and after they reach a certain level blood is removed from the horse's jugular vein. The blood is then separated and the immune blood serum (containing the immune bodies that have been made by the cells) is injected into the animal that is being treated.

Passive immunity occurs as soon as an animal is injected but immune blood serum does not cause the production of antibodies. For this reason passive immunity lasts only 3–6 weeks and ends as soon as the immune bodies that have been injected are eliminated from the animal's body.

Immune blood serums are used for temporary protection against outbreaks of disease. When intended to cure a disease they are injected intravenously; when the use is preventative the injection is made intramuscularly or subcutaneously.

Active immunity is slower to develop and takes 1–2 weeks after an injection is given. However, the effect lasts longer as body cells make their own antibodies (immune bodies) over a longer period when stimulated directly by an infection.

Many times an animal will receive a combined injection of immune blood serum and vaccine in order to give both immediate and long-term protection against an infectious disease. This combination allows a larger level of vaccine to be injected than normal, speeding up immune body production. A common example of just such a combination is the virus-serum innoculation against hog cholera.

Common Factors which Cause Disease

Whenever an animal's defenses are overcome by attacking pathogenic organisms the animal is considered infected (contaminated with disease-producing organisms or matter). But the infection is usually not the only cause of the disease. Several factors may work together to cause the animal's illness (which can also be looked at as an insufficient production of antibodies).

Body defenses are weakened by cold weather, too much work, not enough and/or not the right kind of feed, and by being shipped long distances. Another cause is chronic infection; that is, an infection that lasts a long time or recurs frequently.

Chronic infections and parasites actually make animals more susceptible to other diseases. It works like this: when fighting one kind of microorganism the animal's condition is weakened, and when it's attacked by a second infection it may not be able to produce enough antibodies quickly enough to defend itself. This secondary infection may be caused by microorganisms that invade the body or by ones that are already present without doing any harm until the body's defenses are lowered and they attack.

This is the reason that two diseases often occur at the same time or one right after another. Therefore, when attempting to cure a disease make sure you identify and eliminate all of its contributing factors.

Disease Carriers and Reservoirs

A disease carrier is an animal that carries an infection within its body but doesn't show any of the signs of the illness. This is dangerous because its secretions, feces or urine (depending on the disease) may from time to time contain the infectious organisms and other animals may thus be infected by contact with such secretions. Or, through one or more of the contributing factors to disease (as mentioned previously) the animal itself may be attacked by the infection. It is also possible that the carrier may spread the infection to a normal animal via an insect bite.

Foot-and-mouth disease (FMD) is one of the most dangerous and costly diseases that is spread by carrier animals. A few animals that have been infected with and recovered from the virus that produces the disease maintain a certain quantity of the active virus within their bodies for months and possibly years afterward. From time to time they eliminate this active virus in a high enough proportion to infect other animals.

Reservoir animals—usually wild, undomesticated animals and birds—serve as a constant source of infection to other species through insect bites. A good example of a disease spread via reservoir animals, in this case pigeons and ring-necked pheasants, is equine encephalomyelitis. This is a virus that attacks the brain and spinal cord of equines (horses, mules, and burros) either killing them in a few days, or, if they survive, oftentimes leaving them with permanent brain damage. It's believed that infected birds are bitten by mosquitoes which then transmit the disease to any susceptible equine they subsequently bite.

2

BACTERIA AND VIRUSES

Bacteria

Bacteria are tiny one-celled microorganisms. Depending on their type they can be harmful (disease producing), harmless, or beneficial. The beneficial kind aid in changing the composition of different substances. For instance, they create the process of fermentation needed to make vinegar and to ripen cheese.

The harmful bacteria are divided into three types depending on their shape. Bacilli are rod-shaped; they cause tuberculosis and tetanus. Cocci are round or oval; they cause pneumonia, several forms of mastitis, and many other diseases. Spirilla are shaped like threads or corkscrews; they have been linked to cow and ewe abortions.

Under special conditions some bacteria produce spores which are a resting stage of the microorganism. Spores are very resistant to heat, cold, disinfectants, and poisons. They can live for many years in this dormant (inactive) stage until conditions once again become suitable for them to change back to their prior form. This is why some spore-carried diseases, such as anthrax, may reappear after a lapse of many years in an area where they were thought to have been wiped out.

Some pathogenic bacteria make very strong poisonous substances known as *soluble toxins*. These poisons dissolve in the environment in which the bacteria live—the animal's body. Tetanus and diphtheria, severe infectious diseases, especially of young calves, that kill through blood poisoning, are two diseases caused by bacteria that produce soluble toxins.

Other bacteria carry toxins inside their bodies; these poisons are called *endotoxins*. They are not as strong as soluble toxins. When these types of bacteria die or disintegrate their endotoxins are released and attack certain kinds of tissue cells.

Certain bacteria cause tissue inflammation in the part of the body they attack. Inflammation occurs when a body tissue reacts to infection, injury, or irritation. Its symptoms are redness, pain, swelling, heat, and sometimes loss of function.

Abscesses, swollen cavities where pus collects, are one kind of tissue inflammation caused by these bacteria. Depending on how strong the bacteria are and the ability of the animal to resist their attack, the abscesses may remain in one spot or the infection may pass into the bloodstream and be carried throughout the animal's body. This is usually very dangerous and may cause the animal to die of septicemia (blood poisoning).

Viruses

Viruses are living organisms that are also considered complex proteins; they are many times smaller than bacteria. They live and reproduce (multiply) within living cells. The antibiotics that we use against bacteria are useless in treating viruses as antibiotics can only circulate in body fluids and don't enter living cells.

Viruses may attack particular tissues, such as those of the brain, spinal cord, nerves, skin, membranes, or internal organs. They cause the following animal diseases: foot-and-mouth disease, equine encephalomyelitis, rabies, hog cholera, fowlpox, and many more.

One of the big problems with some viral infections is that they create the proper conditions by which bacteria already present in an animal's body attack it as well. These bacteria are called *secondary bacterial invaders*. They may commonly be present in the animal's body without injuring it or may be responsible for a low-level infection that has little effect. But as soon as certain viruses attack the animal, lowering its natural defenses, these secondary bacterial invaders attack as well. This may be quite serious because the effect of one often increases the strength of the other. This happens frequently in distemper of dogs and horses, hog cholera, swine influenza (hog flu), and other viral diseases.

3

BODY TEMPERATURE

An animal's temperature is an indication of its state of health. If you know the average body temperature and its normal variation by species you can get a good idea of the health of your animals by taking their temperatures once a day. Since fever, an unusually high body temperature, is one of the first and best signs of an infectious disease, taking temperatures can help you diagnose illness.

Temperature can be thought of as a balance between heat that is produced and lost. Both animals and humans produce heat by burning stored energy in the form of fat. The amount of heat that is produced is increased by work, shivering, or an overactive thyroid (the gland that regulates body growth and processes). Animals that feed entirely on plants, such as horses, cattle, and sheep, are also able to produce heat through bacterial fermentation in their stomachs and intestines.

Heat is lost by evaporation of the water vapor in our breath, from the sweat we secrete, and it radiates from our skin when it's warmer than the air around it. Different species lose heat in different ways: pigs have no sweat glands and must roll in mud or water to lower their body temperatures; rabbits, on the other hand, lose heat through their ears.

Normal Temperature Variation

Healthy animals have a higher body temperature during the day than during the night. The variation in large animals, such as horses, mules and cattle, is around 1°F. Very small animals may vary 5–10°F (1.5–7°C) between day and night.

Body temperatures may rise from work, being excited and from long exposure to warm and/or humid weather. If an animal is overheated and can't lower its body temperature quickly enough its normal functions are going to suffer. When this happens to cattle they eat less, lose weight, and produce a smaller than normal quantity of milk.

The most important natural remedy for this problem is water. Heat loss and water loss occur at the same time. An overheated animal that is dehydrated (having lost most of its water) is not able to sweat, which would lower its body temperature, and it may come down with a fever. Again, the best treatment is water. Animals need access to a constant supply of clean, fresh drinking water and must be allowed to drink when they want to!

Temperatures also vary according to the season of the year, by an animal's age and, in the female, in relation to her reproductive cycle. In the cold or winter season, temperatures (measured in the anus) are 1-2°F (.6-1.2°C) lower than in summer.

Young animals show greater day-night temperature differences than older ones. When animals are young and get an infection their temperatures go up much higher than when they are old. In fact, when they are very old and become sick their body temperatures may not change at all.

Before a female ovulates (releasing an egg which the male may then fertilize with his sperm) her temperature usually drops 1°F below the level of the past few days. Then, when she comes into heat, and will allow the male to mount her, her temperature is a little higher than normal. If she becomes pregnant this level will last through the first half of the pregnancy, after which time it drops to normal.

What Is Fever?

Fever is the term used to describe an uncommonly high body temperature. There are several kinds: daytime fever, which may occur as a result of chronic infection, fever caused by an acute infection, and intermittent fever.

In daytime fever the animal's temperature rises a few degrees above the regular daytime level and drops to normal at night. When an animal has an acute infection, both day and nighttime temperatures will be above normal for a few days. Intermittent fevers are caused by long-lasting or frequently recurring diseases, such as brucellosis—a reproductive disease of cattle. The telltale symptom of intermittent fever is an abnormally high body temperature for a few days, then a normal one for several days, and finally the process repeats itself.

A good sign of the onset of fever is a chill. Animals become easily annoyed, they shiver and look for a warm place to curl up in to try and reduce the amount of heat their bodies are giving off. If an animal is chilled its temperature is already above normal; as it shivers it creates more heat and its body temperature goes even higher. This leads to a fever. You will be able to tell that an animal has fever if its rectal temperature is 2°F (1.1°C) higher than the normal highest figure given for that animal in the table, "Normal Temperature Range," on p. 10.

Fever causes a disruption of body processes. Within both the animal and human body the balance between salt and water in the body fluids must be maintained in a stable way so that the body is able to function correctly. If the animal loses too much water, and becomes dehydrated, its body temperature will rise.

A long-lasting fever will cause the animal to lose salt, again disturbing the water-salt balance in body fluids. Signs of this are muscular twitching and even convulsions, if too much salt has been lost. Convulsions, like shivering, produce a lot of heat. They can be stopped by the intravenous (IV) injection of barbiturates (sleep inducing drugs). Always follow the manufacturer's instructions as to dosage. The fever should be treated by cooling down the animal with a cold bath or dip of water or alcohol.

Cattle and horses should have constant access to salt, both when the weather is hot and after a fever, in order to make up the amount they will have lost. If any animal's body temperature ever goes 10°F (6°C) over its normal level it's an indication that it will die soon afterward.

Taking Your Animal's Temperature

An animal's body temperature is taken by inserting a mercury thermometer into its rectum. The thermometer is a glass tube with a thin hollow center and bulb at the bottom filled with mercury, a metal that acts like a liquid at normal temperatures. Large animals take a 5-inch thermometer, small animals a 4-inch one (see Figure 1a).

As the bulb heats up, mercury will rise in the tube. Once it reaches the point that corresponds to the temperature it has been heated to, the mercury remains there. In this way it is easily read. After taking a temperature the thermometer is shaken down, in order to return the mercury to the bulb, and then washed.

First, check to see that the thermometer has been shaken down. If not, do so. Then lubricate it with petroleum jelly or cooking oil and put it bulb first into the animal's rectum as far as it will go. Of course, leave enough of the end sticking out to remove it. Leave the thermometer in at least three minutes (see Figure 1b).

NORMAL TEMPERATURE RANGE

Animal	Temperature Variation (in degrees Fahrenheit)	Average Temperature (in degrees Fahrenheit)
Horse	99–100.8	99.8
Beef cow	101.8–102.4	102
Dairy cow	100.4–102.8	101.5
Sheep	100.9–103.8	102.3
Goat	101.7–105.3	103.8
Pig	101.6–103.6	102.5
Adult chicken, turkey, duck, or goose	105–109.4	107.1
Young chicken, turkey, duck, or goose	102–106	
Rabbit	101.5–103.5	102.5

It is a good idea to tie up cattle, horses, and mules securely when taking their temperatures as they often kick and may injure themselves. Small animals can be restrained by hand.

Get into the habit of taking temperatures at least once daily and writing them down. It will help you discover feverish and infected animals, will aid in the diagnosis of disease, and will give you an idea of how well treatment is working.

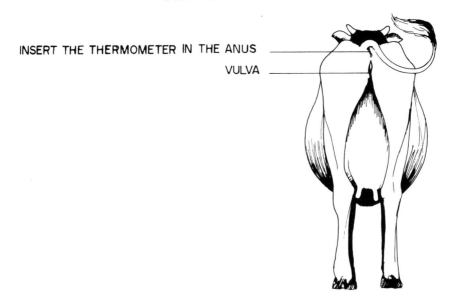

INSERT THE THERMOMETER IN THE ANUS ———
VULVA ———

Figure 1a.   How to take an animal's temperature.

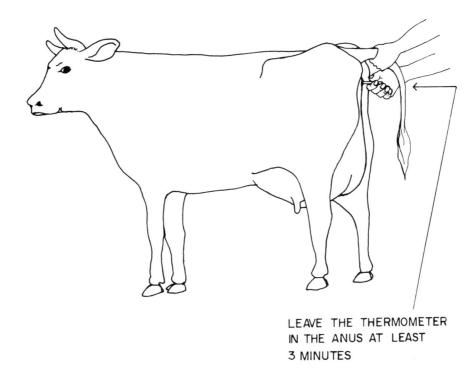

LEAVE THE THERMOMETER
IN THE ANUS AT LEAST
3 MINUTES

Figure 1b.   How to take an animal's temperature.

4

WEIGHING ANIMALS

The dosage of veterinary drugs and biological products is figured per pound multiplied by an animal's total body weight. Buyers and sellers need to calculate animal weights in order to fix prices and conduct their business. Breeders must also be able to compare weights of different animals at the same stages of their lives in order to properly select future breeding stock.

Large commercial scales are usually in short supply. But with only a tape measure and several simple formulas you can estimate your animal's weight fairly accurately.

Horses

The "Horse Weight Table" (p. 14-15) was prepared by Dr. José Serrano Pinto of the School of Veterinary Medicine, Bogotá, Colombia.

To find the weight of your horse measure, using a tape measure, these three places: 1) around the chest just behind the shoulders, 2) around the abdomen, and 3) a straight line between the hipbone and the middle of the shoulder (see Figure 2).

Add these measurements together. Then look down the column entitled The Sum of the Measurements until you find your horse's total or the number closest to it. The figure in the next column to the right, Corresponding Weight, will tell you how much your horse weighs.

Dairy Cows

The weight table for dairy cows was prepared from research done by H. P. Davis and R. F. Morgan of the University of Nebraska. It is easier to use than the horse weight table because only one measurement is

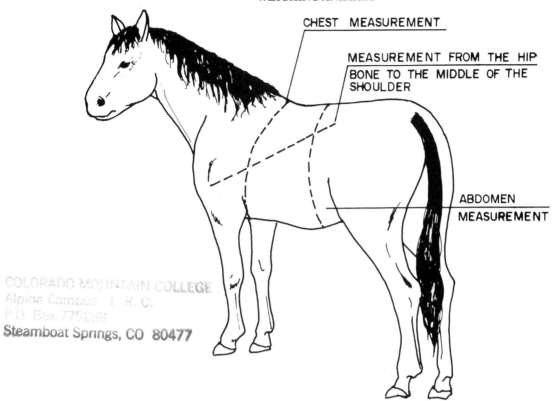

Figure 2.   Measurements to determine the weight of a horse.

made: around the chest just behind the shoulders. Pull the tape tightly around the chest without pinching skin or flesh and take your reading (see Figure 3).

After finding the cow's chest measurement, check across in the weight column under the animal's breed. If your animal is of a mixed breed choose the breed it most closely resembles. Then measure several animals of the same type and see how much their weights vary from those given in the table. Average their weight variation and either add or subtract it from the weight given in the table of the breed your cow most closely resembles.

For example, you have five mixed-breed cows that most closely resemble Holsteins. However, with the same chest measurements as pureblood Holsteins the total of the difference of their weights is 50 pounds less than those given in the table. Since you have five animals, the average weight variation is 50 divided by 5, or 10 pounds per cow less than an average Holstein. So your Holstein-type cow that has a chest measurement of 63 inches will weigh approximately 728 – 10 = 718 pounds (using the "Dairy Cow Weight Table" on p. 16-17). This is an average figure.

In order to be more accurate, it's important to mention one additional point: this table is correct to within 7 percent of an animal's total weight. What this means is that an animal will weigh between 7 percent less and 7 percent more than the given figure.

Let's go back to the last example. We have determined that your mixed-breed cow weighs 718 pounds. Seven percent of 718 is 50.26 (.07 × 718 = 50.26).   So your animal actually weighs somewhere

HORSE WEIGHT TABLE

The Sum of the Measurements (in inches)	Corresponding Weight (in pounds)	The Sum of the Measurements (in inches)	Corresponding Weight (in pounds)	The Sum of the Measurements (in inches)	Corresponding Weight (in pounds)
114.96	226.6	138.19	369.6	161.81	644.6
115.35	226.6	138.58	369.6	162.60	651.2
116.14	228.8	138.98	374.0	163.00	655.6
116.54	231.0	139.37	374.0	163.39	660.0
116.93	233.2	140.16	378.4	164.17	664.4
117.32	235.4	140.55	382.8	164.57	668.8
118.11	237.6	140.94	382.8	164.96	673.2
118.50	239.8	142.13	387.2	165.35	677.6
118.90	239.8	142.52	391.6	166.14	682.0
119.69	242.0	142.91	396.0	166.54	686.4
120.08	244.2	144.49	400.4	166.93	690.8
120.47	244.2	144.88	404.8	167.32	695.2
120.87	248.6	145.67	413.6	168.11	701.8
121.65	253.0	146.06	422.4	168.50	708.4
122.05	257.4	146.46	435.6	168.90	712.8
122.44	259.6	146.85	435.6	169.69	717.2
122.83	261.8	147.64	444.4	170.08	723.8
123.62	264.0	148.03	448.8	170.47	730.4
124.02	264.0	148.42	457.6	170.87	739.2
124.41	266.2	148.82	466.4	171.65	748.0
125.20	268.4	149.61	473.0	172.83	765.6
125.60	268.4	150.00	477.4	173.62	770.0
125.98	270.6	150.39	477.4	174.02	774.4
126.77	272.8	151.18	488.4	174.41	778.8
127.16	275.0	151.57	497.2	175.20	783.2
127.56	281.6	151.97	506.0	175.60	792.0
127.95	286.0	152.36	519.2	175.98	798.6
128.35	290.4	152.76	528.0	176.38	803.0
128.74	294.8	153.15	532.4	177.17	814.0
129.53	294.8	153.54	541.2	177.56	822.8
129.92	299.2	153.94	545.6	177.95	831.6
130.31	299.2	154.33	550.0	178.35	833.8
131.10	308.0	155.12	554.4	179.13	836.0
131.50	312.4	155.51	561.0	179.53	840.4
131.89	316.8	155.91	572.0	179.92	842.6
132.68	321.2	156.69	576.4	180.31	847.0
133.07	325.6	157.09	580.8	181.10	858.0
133.46	330.0	157.48	589.6	181.50	866.8
133.86	334.4	157.87	598.4	181.89	875.6
134.65	338.8	158.66	607.2	182.68	880.0
135.04	341.0	159.06	611.8	183.07	886.6
135.43	345.4	159.45	616.0	183.46	893.2
135.83	352.0	159.84	618.2	183.86	897.6
136.61	356.4	160.63	624.8	184.65	904.2
137.01	360.8	161.02	633.6	185.04	908.6
137.40	365.2	161.42	638.0	185.43	915.2

The Sum of the Measurements (in inches)	Corresponding Weight (in pounds)	The Sum of the Measurements (in inches)	Corresponding Weight (in pounds)
185.83	924.0	200.00	1,188.0
186.61	928.4	200.39	1,199.0
187.01	932.8	201.97	1,245.2
187.40	941.6	202.36	1,258.4
188.19	954.8	203.15	1,276.0
188.58	963.6	203.54	1,293.6
188.98	974.6	203.94	1,311.2
189.37	981.2	204.33	1,320.0
190.16	990.0	205.12	1,328.8
190.55	998.8	205.51	1,346.4
190.94	1,009.8	205.91	1,364.0
191.34	1,018.6	206.69	1,381.6
192.13	1,029.6	207.09	1,399.2
192.52	1,038.4	207.48	1,412.4
192.91	1,047.2	207.87	1,430.0
193.31	1,056.0	208.66	1,447.6
194.09	1,064.8	209.06	1,456.4
194.49	1,073.6	209.45	1,469.6
194.88	1,082.4	209.84	1,478.4
195.67	1,095.6	210.63	1,491.6
196.06	1,104.4	211.02	1,504.8
196.46	1,117.6	211.42	1,518.0
196.85	1,130.8	211.81	1,531.2
197.64	1,144.0	212.60	1,540.0
198.03	1,157.2	213.00	1,548.8
198.43	1,166.0	213.39	1,553.2
198.82	1,172.6	214.17	1,557.6
199.61	1,179.2	214.57	1,562.0

between 667.74 pounds (718 − 50.26 = 667.74) and 768.26 pounds (718 + 50.26 = 768.26). But for a good average we can say your cow weighs 718 pounds.

Pigs

Pig weights are determined using this easy formula:

$$\text{Weight} = \frac{\text{Chest Girth} \times \text{Chest Girth} \times \text{Length}}{400}$$

Chest girth is figured by passing the tape measure around the pig's chest just behind the shoulders. Length is measured from a point between the ears to the beginning of the tail (see Figure 4). If the pig weighs less than 150 pounds add 7 pounds to the final figure you get from the formula.

DAIRY COW WEIGHT TABLE
Live Weight (in pounds)

Chest Girth (in inches)	Holstein	Jersey	Guernsey	Ayrshire	Average
21	—	32	—	—	—
22	—	37	—	—	—
23	46	42	38	38	41
24	51	47	43	43	46
25	57	52	48	49	52
26	64	59	54	54	58
27	71	65	61	61	64
28	78	72	67	67	71
29	86	80	74	74	78
30	95	88	82	82	87
31	104	97	90	90	95
32	113	106	99	99	104
33	123	115	108	108	114
34	134	125	118	118	124
35	145	136	129	128	135
36	156	147	140	139	146
37	169	159	151	150	157
38	181	172	163	162	170
39	195	185	176	175	183
40	209	199	190	188	196
41	224	213	204	202	211
42	239	228	219	216	226
43	255	244	234	231	241
44	272	260	250	247	257
45	289	277	267	264	274
46	307	295	285	281	292
47	326	314	304	299	311
48	345	333	323	317	330
49	365	353	343	337	350
50	386	373	364	357	370
51	408	395	385	378	392
52	430	417	407	400	414
53	453	440	431	422	436
54	477	464	455	446	460
55	502	489	480	470	485
56	527	515	506	495	511
57	553	541	532	521	537
58	580	568	560	548	564
59	608	597	589	575	592
60	637	626	618	604	621
61	667	655	648	633	651
62	697	686	680	664	682
63	728	718	712	695	713
64	761	751	746	727	746
65	794	784	780	760	780
66	828	819	815	794	814
67	863	855	852	830	850
68	899	891	889	866	886
69	935	929	928	903	924

DAIRY COW WEIGHT TABLE
Live Weight (in pounds)

Chest Girth (in inches)	Holstein	Jersey	Guernsey	Ayrshire	Average
70	973	967	968	941	962
71	1012	1007	1009	981	1002
72	1052	1048	1050	1021	1043
73	1092	1089	1093	1062	1084
74	1134	1132	1137	1104	1127
75	1177	1176	1183	1148	1171
76	1220	1221	1229	1193	1216
77	1265	1267	1277	1239	1262
78	1311	1314	1326	1285	1309
79	1357	1362	1376	1333	1357
80	1405	1412	1427	1383	1407
81	1454	1463	1480	1433	1458
82	1504	1514	1534	1484	1509
83	1555	—	1589	1538	—
84	1607	—	—	1592	—
85	1660	—	—	1647	—
86	1715	—	—	1703	—
87	1760	—	—	—	—
88	1827	—	—	—	—
89	1884	—	—	—	—
90	1942	—	—	—	—
91	2002	—	—	—	—
92	2064	—	—	—	—
93	2127	—	—	—	—
94	2190	—	—	—	—
95	2254	—	—	—	—

For example, your pig measures 39 inches around the chest and 42 inches in length.

$$\text{The pig's weight} = \frac{39 \times 39 \times 42}{400}$$

$$= \frac{63,882}{400}$$

$$= 157.2 \text{ pounds}$$

However, if you have a young pig that measures 30 inches around the chest and 32 inches in length the formula looks like this:

$$\text{The pig's weight} = \frac{30 \times 30 \times 32}{400}$$

$$= \frac{28,800}{400}$$

$$= 72 \text{ pounds}$$

$$+ \ 7 \text{ pounds} \quad \text{(72 is less than 150 so you must add 7 pounds to the total)}$$

The pig's true weight = 79 pounds

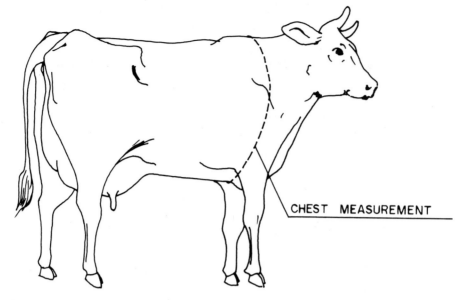

CHEST MEASUREMENT

Figure 3.   Measurements to determine the weight of a dairy cow.

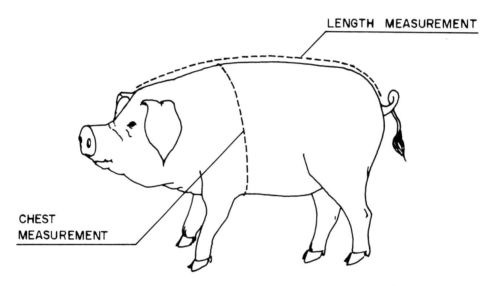

LENGTH MEASUREMENT

CHEST
MEASUREMENT

Figure 4.   Measurements to determine the weight of a pig.

5

ANIMAL SPECIMENS FOR LABORATORY ANALYSIS

The analysis of animal specimens can be a great help in the diagnosis of disease and prescription of drug treatment. The main reason for analysis is to determine exactly which disease or diseases an animal suffers from. This is oftentimes important in order to treat the animal and its herdmates, who have also been exposed to the same infection. We also need this information to start with preventive measures to ensure that the conditions that gave rise to the disease are removed.

Samples of blood and fecal matter can be taken from living animals that suffer from a chronic or slowly developing disease. If the animal shows signs of acute disease it's best to treat it right away based on a diagnosis of the available symptoms. Then if there is any uncertainty as to what disease it's affected by, specimens should be taken and sent to a laboratory for analysis. This is not only done to be certain of how to treat the animal but also to decide what preventive steps must be taken to protect its herdmates. For the same reason, specimens of animals that have died of disease should be collected and analyzed.

Blood

Blood is taken from an animal to determine what infectious disease it's suffering from. First, sterilize two glass jars by boiling them at least ten minutes in water. Let them dry completely on clean unused paper towels or toilet paper. Next, extract 10–20 cubic centimeters of blood from the jugular vein and put it into one of the dry sterilized jars. The best kind of jar is one with a rubber or plastic top. (Any kind of metal will react with the blood, which you don't want to happen.)

Leave the jar in a slightly inclined position for a few hours. The blood serum (a clear yellowish fluid) will separate from the coagulated blood corpuscles (a deep red color). Pour the serum into the second dry sterilized jar, making sure none of the coagulate passes with it. Firmly put the top on the jar and label it with your name and address, the date, and some way of identifying the animal from which it was taken.

In the event of a suspected case of anthrax all you have to do is soak a piece of chalk, clean dry paper, or cotton with the animal's blood and put it in a dry, sterilized jar or plastic bag. Make sure the top of the jar is screwed on tightly or, if you use a plastic bag, that it's tied securely and placed inside of a second dry, sterilized bag that has been tied as well.

Fecal Matter

Samples of excrement can be analyzed to tell which parasites an animal suffers from. A portion of fresh feces the size of a chicken's egg is put into a sterilized glass jar or one plastic bag is put inside of another (for protection in case the first breaks). Samples must be fresh and be delivered to the laboratory for analysis as soon as possible.

Body Tissue

When an animal dies of a disease it's a good idea to know why, especially considering the economic value of the rest of the herd and the danger of it being infected with the same disease. The animal must be dissected and small sections taken from organs such as the liver, kidney, brain, etc. These tissue samples are generally 1 inch high × 1 inch long × ¼ inch wide.

Always wear plastic gloves and rubber boots when dissecting an animal that has died from an unknown cause. After finishing the dissection and before leaving the site, disinfect all tools and knives, and the plastic gloves and rubber boots you wore. You must remember to wash yourself thoroughly after such an operation.

If the carcass is thought to contain infectious microorganisms before beginning the dissection, you should stuff the anus, vagina, mouth, and nostrils with clean towels or rags to absorb body fluids. These must later be burned.

Each tissue sample is put into its own sterilized wide-mouth glass jar. Each jar is then filled with one-half boiled, sterile water and one-half glycerine. The top is firmly closed and sealed, and delivered to a laboratory as soon as possible. If for some reason you can't get them to a lab right away, put them in the freezer until you are able to deliver them.

Information

Regardless of whether you personally go to the laboratory to drop off a specimen or send it in the mail, you must include certain information with it. The following is a suggested list of data that should be included with your sample:

1. Your name, address, and the date
2. Type of animal and breed
3. Animal's sex and age
4. What samples have been taken
5. The suspected disease
6. The physical symptoms
7. Whether or not the animal suffered from the same or a similar disease previously
8. If so, describe treatment and length of time taken for disease to recur
9. Whether or not the disease symptoms are common in the area
10. List animal's vaccinations, with dates.

6

DRENCHING

Pouring a liquid down an animal's throat is called *drenching*. It's usually done to administer awful tasting medicines that must be given orally and those which an animal refuses to eat mixed in feed, or refuses to drink mixed in water.

Drenching must be done slowly, very carefully, and with an understanding of what happens inside the animal's body during the procedure. I will use the cow as an example.

As with all animals and humans, the back part of a cow's throat has two tubes leading from it—the windpipe and the esophagus. The windpipe brings air from the nostrils and mouth to the lungs. While the animal is breathing in or out, the inlet to the windpipe is wide open. When the animal swallows, the inlet closes.

The esophagus, the tube that brings food and liquid to the cow's stomach, is always closed as the cow breathes. However, as soon as the cow swallows, the esophagus opens up and the windpipe closes.

A serious problem occurs when an animal doesn't want to swallow something it's being forced to swallow. This is where you must be very careful when drenching. When food or liquid is forced down a cow's throat and it doesn't swallow of its own free will, the windpipe remains open and the esophagus stays shut. Thus, the food or liquid passes into the windpipe.

Two things can happen: If solid food enters the windpipe the cow could possibly choke to death as its air supply is blocked off. If liquid enters the windpipe, the cow could choke if its head isn't lowered quickly enough to allow it to cough out the fluid. Even if it is able to cough it out chances are good the cow will come down with pneumonia and become very sick, if not die. So take your time and be careful when you drench an animal!

Drenching Directions

First, put a rubber or plastic hose on the end of a plastic bottle, like those that detergent comes in, or a long-necked glass bottle. This is so the cow doesn't accidentally break the glass and injure itself (see Figure 5).

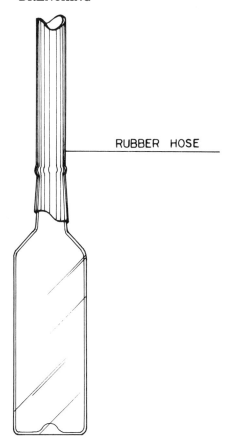

Figure 5. Drenching bottle and hose.

Put your thumb and first finger into the cow's nostrils and hold them firmly. Force up on the nostrils in order to raise the animal's head a little so the liquid will run gently from the bottle into its mouth and toward its throat.

The rubber hose is put into the cow's mouth from the side with your other hand. The end of it is placed on the back part of the center of the tongue. (See if you can manage this by yourself, but it may be a two-person operation.)

The liquid is poured slowly from the bottle when the animal has its mouth closed. You must frequently stop pouring in order to let the cow swallow. What you are really trying to do in drenching is make an animal simulate its own natural drinking style. If a cow coughs while being drenched immediately lower its head so it can expel the liquid that has entered its windpipe.

Horses are drenched just like cattle, but sheep require much more care than either. When drenching sheep you should make sure they are standing on firm, level ground. Also, their noses must never be raised any higher than their eyes or they might strangle. Give a liquid drench to sheep more slowly than you would to either cattle or horses.

If any of the animals you drench doesn't drink the liquid you've just poured into its mouth stop pouring and strongly massage the length of its throat and neck. That usually does the trick. If it doesn't, lower the animal's head, wait for it to expel or cough out the medicine, and then start over again.

Awful tasting liquids don't taste any better when they are forcibly poured down an animal's throat, nor is the cow going to appreciate having its head held up by you grasping its nostrils. The animal's normal reaction is to fight back by shaking its head and by pulling back and away from you or to the side. It's quite possible you will get thrown around (now you see why we put a rubber hose on the bottle) and an easy job could become a lot of trouble.

A simple solution is to take a rope and double it in the middle. Pass the two ends through the loop and you've got a noose (see Figures 6A and B). Put the noose over the cow's upper jaw and slip it toward the back part of the mouth. Now draw it tight and tie the loose ends to a tree limb or a projecting wooden beam on your barn or other building (see Figure 7). Make sure the cow's head is raised only slightly and that the knot can be released quickly in case the animal starts to cough and choke!

A good trick for drenching a calf if you are alone is to straddle it as if you were riding it. Squeeze its neck and head between your legs, but not too hard or you might choke it (see Figure 8).

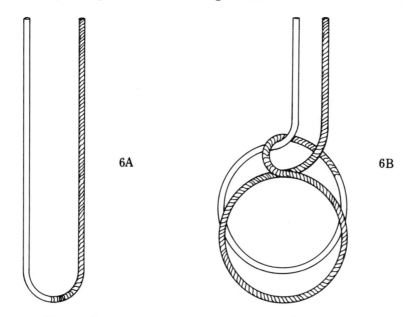

6A   6B

Figure 6.   How to tie a noose.

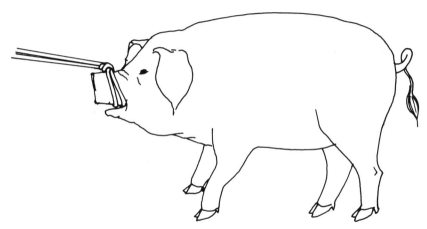

Figure 7.   Using the noose.

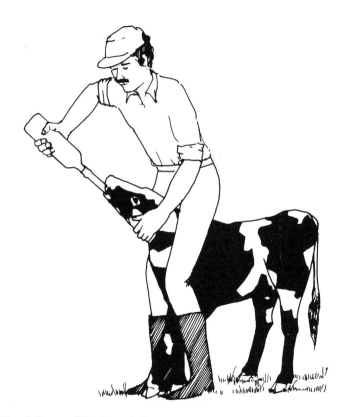

Figure 8.   Straddle a calf to drench it.

7

SYRINGES

A hypodermic syringe is an instrument with a needle attached to one end, with which drugs, medicines, and biological products are injected into or under the skin. Animals are also given medicines by way of the mouth, but injection through the skin usually works better because the medication affects the animal more rapidly than with the other methods. Injected medication does not pass through the digestive tract, and it is therefore not mixed, diluted, or chemically altered by food, water, saliva, or digestive secretions, so smaller amounts are needed.

However, because the injection is made under the skin you are opening a route for germs to enter. For this reason the injection must be made under the cleanest possible conditions. There are many different kinds of injections. They vary according to the condition that you are treating or trying to prevent, the intended effect on the animal, and what quantity and type of product is to be injected. Depending on the type of animal, the same kind of shot may be given in a different part of the body (see Chapter 8, Types of Injections).

After you have selected the spot where the injection will be made, all hair or fur around the immediate area must first be clipped with a pair of scissors or clippers and then shaved off with a razor or sharp knife. The bare skin is left exposed.

The injection site is then washed with soap and warm water to remove dirt, dust, and feces. After drying with a paper towel or clean, unused toiletpaper, the spot is swabbed with a piece of sterile cotton dipped in an antiseptic (a substance such as alcohol that represses the action of microorganisms).

The entire syringe is disassembled and all the needles you will use need to be sterilized by boiling in water for 5–10 minutes. Several paper towels or unused sheets of toiletpaper are placed on a flat surface. The syringe parts are tapped against the paper to remove drops of water; needles are blown through. The syringe is then reassembled and laid on the clean paper. Be sure no water remains inside.

It is very important that after being sterilized all needles are kept from coming in contact with anything except the clean paper towels. Otherwise they will no longer be sterile and must be boiled once again. In theory, a new sterilized needle should be used with each animal that will be injected. In laboratory conditions, if you did not have a needle for every animal, you would keep sterilizing the few you did have after each use. However, this is impractical in the barn, out in the field, or on the range. If you must reuse a needle dip it in an antiseptic solution, such as alcohol, after giving each injection. The one exception to this is when injecting live vaccines. Then you must use a newly sterilized needle for each animal and disinfect the injection site with lemon juice—never use a chemical disinfectant.

The point of this is to avoid passing an infection or disease from one animal to another. This could happen quite easily if one animal were sick and the needle you used to inject it with was not disinfected before you used it on the other animals to be treated at the same time. What might have been an isolated case of disease all of a sudden becomes a serious outbreak due to carelessness. Don't let this happen to you—disinfect your needles!

Filling the Syringe

Most bottles of drugs and biological products have a metal cap with a small round piece in the center that must be pried out. When you remove this small piece of metal a rubber top is exposed. Each time before removing solution from the bottle with the needle of your syringe the rubber top should be disinfected by swabbing it with a piece of sterile cotton dipped in alcohol.

Before buying any product make sure that the metal top is intact—this is your guarantee that the product has not been previously used or adulterated since leaving the manufacturer.

There are two ways to fill a syringe: by creating a vacuum in the bottle of solution and by building up pressure inside the bottle. Of the two methods, building up pressure will fill a syringe faster, but both work equally as well.

To use the vacuum method, put a needle on the syringe and push the syringe plunger all the way in. Turn the bottle of solution upside down after having swabbed the rubber top with alcohol. When using live vaccines disinfect the rubber top with lemon juice. Push the needle through the top and slowly pull out the plunger, filling the syringe. Finally, disinfect the needle before giving the injection, and use an unused needle for live vaccines (see Figure 9a and b). To fill a syringe using pressure, proceed as in the vacuum method, but before pushing the needle through the rubber bottle top make sure that the syringe plunger has been pulled all the way out. Push the plunger in a little bit, forcing some air into the bottle. This in turn builds up pressure within the bottle so that when you pull out on the plunger, solution is immediately forced into the syringe. Continue pushing in and pulling out on the plunger until the syringe is full (see Figures 10a to e). Make sure you have disinfected the needle before giving the first injection, but remember that live vaccines are the exception to this rule.

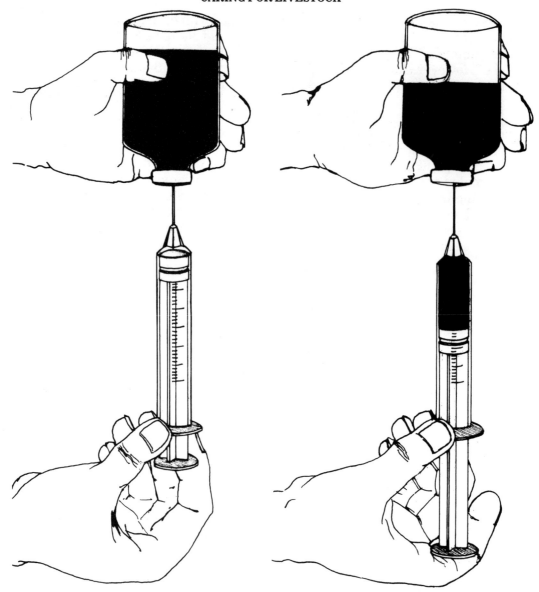

Figure 9a.   **Using vacuum to fill a syringe.**   **Figure 9b.**   **Using vacuum to fill a syringe.**

Checkpoints Before Injecting

1. Is the proper drug or biological product being used for the condition you want to prevent or treat in accordance with the manufacturer's recommendations for species, age, and weight, or in accordance with accepted veterinary practice?
2. Is the drug or biological product being used before the expiration date stamped on the product box or bottle?
3. Is the proper sized syringe and needle being utilized?
4. Have the syringe and needles been sterilized by boiling 5 to 10 minutes? Are there enough sterilized needles for each of the animals to be injected; if not, the needles you do have must be disinfected after each use. When injecting live vaccines use a new sterilized needle for each animal.

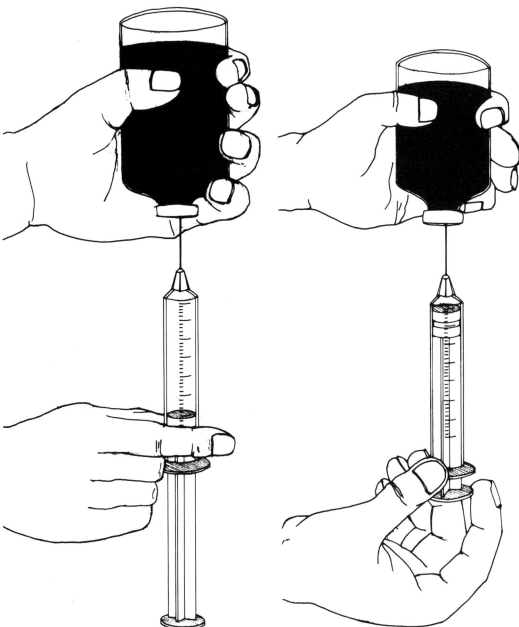

Figure 10a. Using pressure to fill a syringe.   **Figure 10b.** Using pressure to fill a syringe.

5. Be sure no water remains inside the syringe or needle.
6. Has the needle used to remove the solution from its bottle been disinfected before proceeding with the injection? In the case of live vaccines change the needle for a newly sterilized one.
7. Be sure no air, air bubbles, or foam remain inside the syringe once it has been filled. This is extremely important! After the syringe has been filled turn it so the needle angles toward the sky. This will cause air bubbles and foam to rise toward the needle. If you tap the side of the syringe with your fingernail it will speed the process and force the most stubborn bubbles to rise. Slowly push the plunger in until all the bubbles and foam have been expelled.

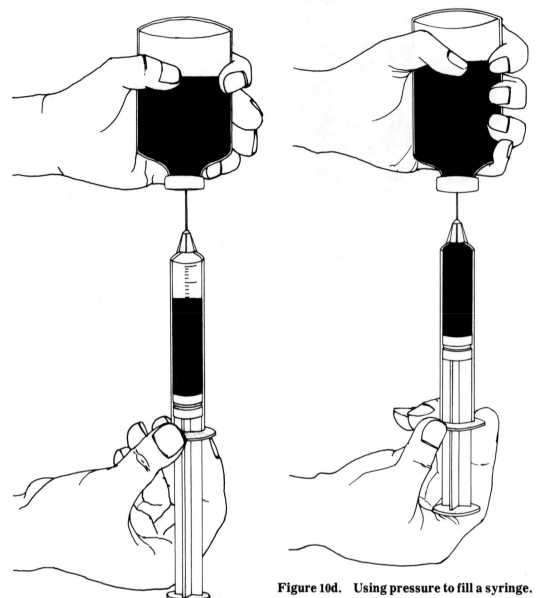

Figure 10d.   Using pressure to fill a syringe.

Figure 10c.   Using pressure to fill a syringe.

If an air bubble is injected into an animal's vein it will pass through the blood system. If it reaches the heart it is possible the animal will die.

8. Have hair and fur been cut from the injection site leaving bare skin? Has the site been washed, dried, and swabbed with alcohol or another disinfectant? When injecting live vaccines disinfect the injection site with lemon juice.

9. Is the right kind of injection being made in the right place in the animal's body?

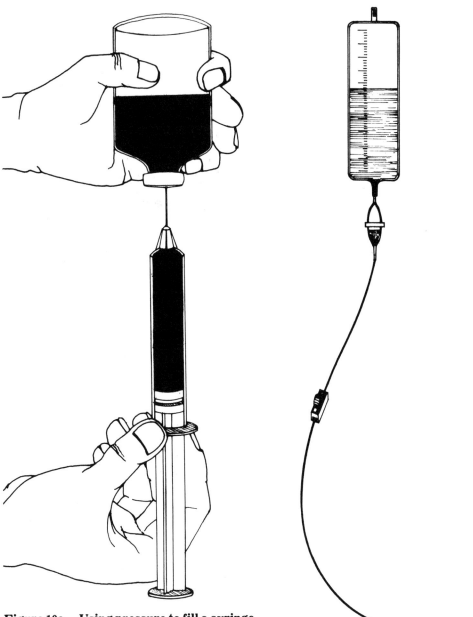

Figure 10e.   Using pressure to fill a syringe.

Figure 11.   An injection outfit.

Kinds of Syringes

Just as there are different kinds of injections, there are different kinds of syringes. Obviously, small animals will be injected with smaller doses than large animals. At times the dose is very tiny, as in the case of chickens, turkeys, ducks, and rabbits, and the indicated syringe must not only be small in size (5-10 cubic centimeters) but with easily read, accurately measured gradations.

But when injecting a bull or horse, or other large animal, a large hypodermic syringe (25–40 cc) is normally used. In cases when a very large amount of solution (greater than 40 cubic centimeters) must be administered, or when the type of medicine would inflame the animal's tissue were any of the other injection methods used, a special syringe called an injection outfit is utilized.

An injection outfit is used to give intravenous and intraperitoneal shots. Intravenous shots are given into veins; intraperitoneal shots are given through the peritoneum, the membrane lining the abdominal cavity. An injection outfit is made of a hollow piece of plastic sharpened at one end that's pushed through the rubber top of the medicine bottle. This holds the solution to be injected upside down and above the animal. The hollow piece of sharpened plastic is connected to a rubber or plastic tube, which holds the needle in its other end. There is no plunger in this type of syringe and the injection is made using gravity. The rate of flow of the solution is controlled by a little plastic adjustment, actually a wheel which holds the tube between itself and its holder, that allows the tube to remain open or squeezes it partially shut depending on the number of cubic centimeters you want to inject per minute (see Figure 11).

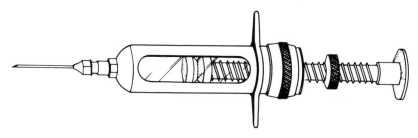

Figure 12a.   Assembled metal syringe.

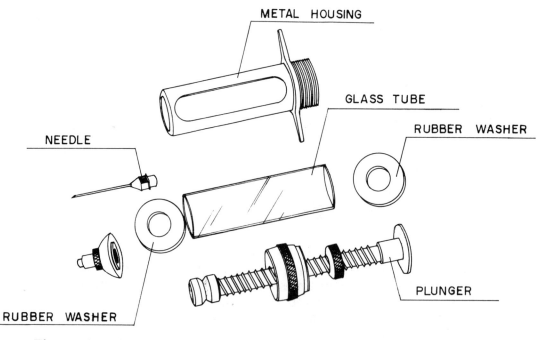

Figure 12b.   Disassembled metal syringe.

Use the kind of syringe that is appropriate for the animal you are injecting and also for the amount of solution to be injected. Syringes are made of metal, glass, and plastic; the only differences between them are how easily and accurately they can be used to inject, considering their size, sturdiness, or fragility of construction, and purchase price (see Figures 12a and b, metal syringe; 13a and b, small plastic syringe; 14a and b, large plastic syringe; 15a and b, glass syringe).

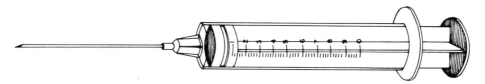

Figure 13a.   Small assembled plastic syringe (for poultry and rabbits).

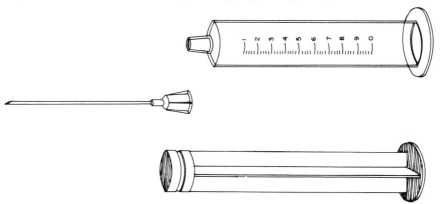

Figure 13b.   Small disassembled plastic syringe.

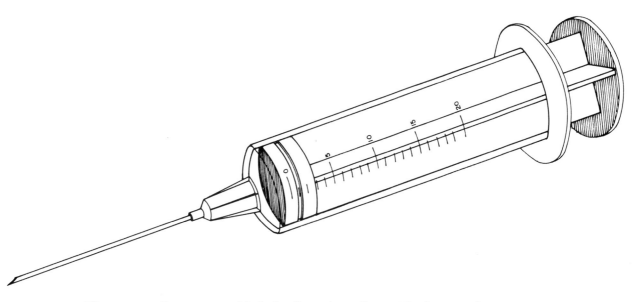

Figure 14a.   Large assembled plastic syringe (for cattle, horses, sheep, goats, and pigs).

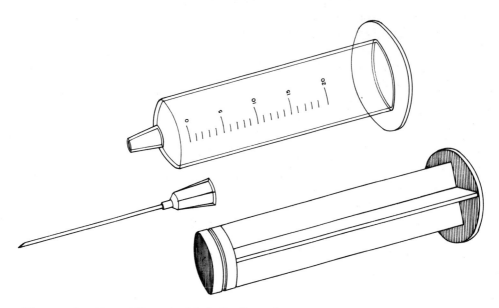

Figure 14b.   Large disassembled plastic syringe.

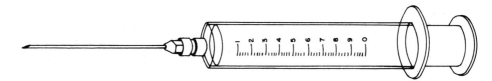

Figure 15a.   Assembled glass syringe (for small animals and poultry).

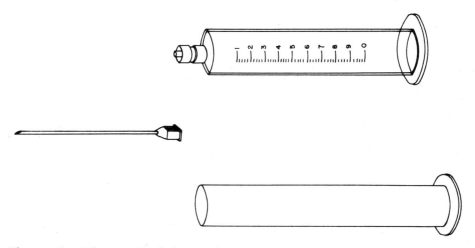

Figure 15b.   Disassembled glass syringe.

8

TYPES OF
INJECTIONS

Before injecting any drug or biological product you must read the manufacturer's instructions to determine what amount should be given according to breed, age, and weight. The instructions will also indicate in what part of the animal's body, and with what kind of technique, the injection should be administered.

Intradermal

An intradermal injection is made into the skin rather than under it, as is the case with all other types of injections. The skin is a very thin tissue made of several layers which serves as the outer covering of the human and animal body. Because it is so thin a very fine-gauge needle is used to fit between the layers. Use a number 19 needle or smaller (the higher the number the smaller the gauge). Make sure the needle is sharp and the injection is done very carefully or you may puncture the skin, making the injection subcutaneous instead of intradermal.

Skin (but no flesh) is pinched between your thumb and forefinger making a 2–3-inch-long ridge. Holding the needle parallel to the mound of skin, insert the whole length. Usually, if it has been inserted properly, the needle lies very close to the surface and you can see it through the few layers of skin that cover it (see Figure 16).

Slowly inject the dose as you withdraw the needle. The solution will fill the needle's track if the injection is done correctly. After removing the needle stick your finger over the hole it made entering the skin and press down. This will keep the solution from leaking out. If the injection was a vaccination the lump left by the solution in the needle's track will grow larger in the next few days (see "How to Give an Intradermal Injection," p. 36–38, Figures 17a, b, and c; Figure 17d indicates where to apply an intradermal injection in cattle, horses, and mules).

35

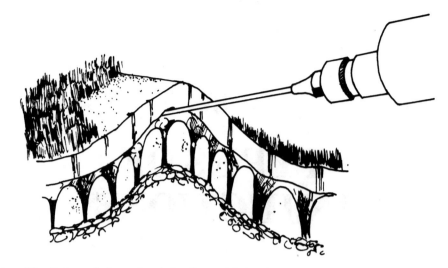

Figure 16.   Internal view of an intradermal injection.

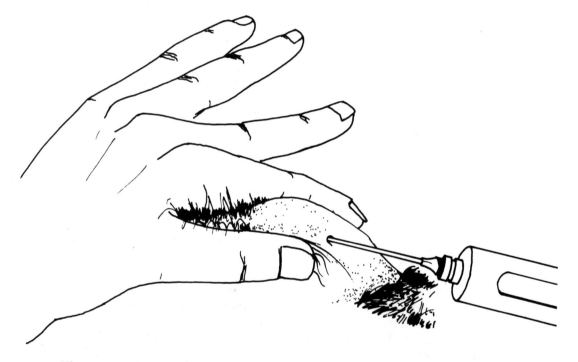

Figure 17a.   How to give an intradermal injection.

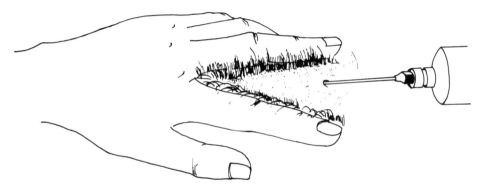

Figure 17b.   How to give an intradermal injection.

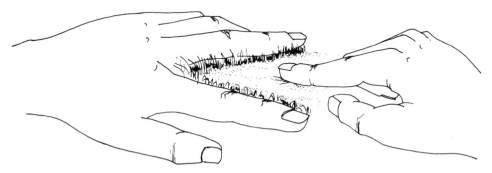

Figure 17c.   How to give an intradermal injection.

Subcutaneous

The subcutaneous injection is made directly below the skin and above the flesh. It differs from the intradermal injection in that the needle penetrates and goes through the skin.

The spot to give this type of shot is where the skin lies loosely. The best places are: in cattle, horses, and mules—the flat part on the side of the neck; pigs—behind the ear; sheep and goats—the front armpit or the upper part of the inside of the hind leg; in fowl—the breast; and in rabbits—the chest or side of the neck.

The animal's skin is pinched between thumb and forefinger, pulling it away from the flesh. The syringe is held perpendicular to the injection site. In one steady motion the needle is pushed through the skin and then turned to the side to keep it from entering the layer of flesh below it.

Next the syringe plunger is pulled out a little to make sure the needle has not been inserted in a vein. If it has you'll be able to tell by the blood that's drawn into the syringe. If you see blood pull the needle out a little and repeat the procedure. If you still see blood remove the needle completely and use another spot to make the injection. This is very important as certain drugs and biological products, when injected into a vein can harm or kill the animal!

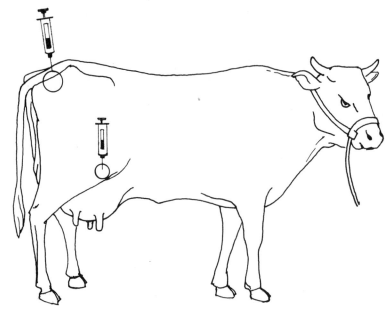

Figure 17d.   Intradermal injection in cattle, horses, and mules.

If no blood appeared when you pulled out slightly on the syringe plunger, make the injection. After completing the injection gently massage the site to aid in the absorption of the solution (see Figures 18—cow; 19—horse; 20a and b—pig; 21a and b—sheep; 22—fowl; 23—rabbit).

Intramuscular

This injection is made into a muscle, usually in the neck or thigh, because they're large and offer many suitable spots. Birds are injected in the thigh or side of the chest.

Small animals should be restrained by a helper; larger ones need to be tied up. Goats and sheep can be held from behind by a helper who grasps the front legs and seats them on their rump (see Figure 24). If that doesn't quiet them, hold them on the ground on their backs.

Animals are usually more frightened of being suddenly pricked with a needle than concerned with the pain it causes them. It's not unusual for them to jump, struggle against their bonds, run off, kick, or bite. Not only does this prevent you from giving the necessary intramuscular shot but it could break the needle off while still in the animal's body, causing further complications. To avoid startling the animal with the needle, tap it hard a couple of times in the injection site, then insert the needle.

The injection is made as follows: pull the skin to the side stretching it tight over the muscle tissue. Insert the needle perpendicularly to the skin and straight through it directly into the muscle. Pull the plunger out

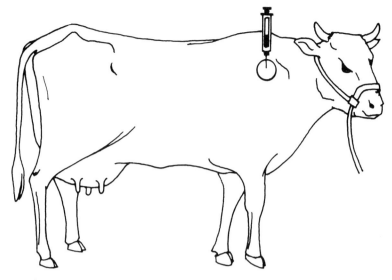

Figure 18.   Subcutaneous injection in the cow.

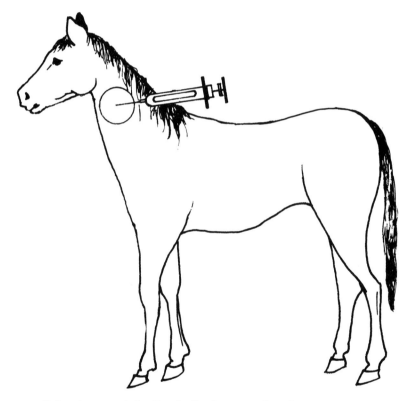

Figure 19.   Subcutaneous injection in the horse and mule.

slightly to check whether the needle is in a vein. If it's not in a vein inject the required amount of solution. Massage the injection site after giving the shot to hasten absorption by the muscle tissue (see Figures 25—cow; 26—horse; 27a and b—pig; 28—sheep; 29—fowl).

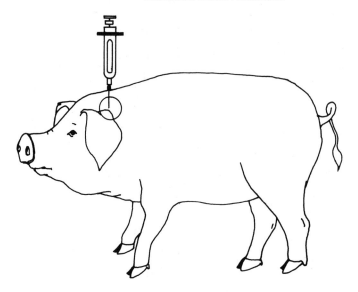

Figure 20a.   Subcutaneous injection in the pig.

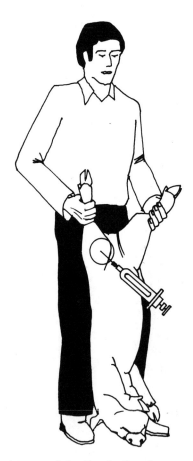

Figure 20b.   Subcutaneous injection in the pig.

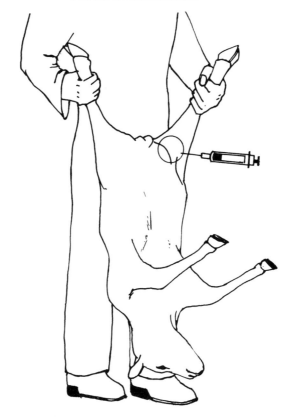

Figure 21a. **Subcutaneous injection in sheep.**

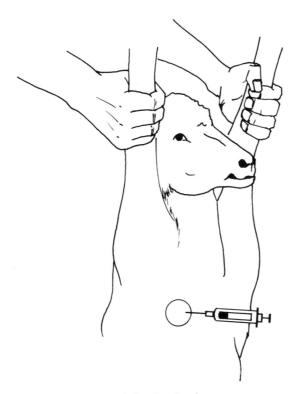

Figure 21b. **Subcutaneous injection in sheep.**

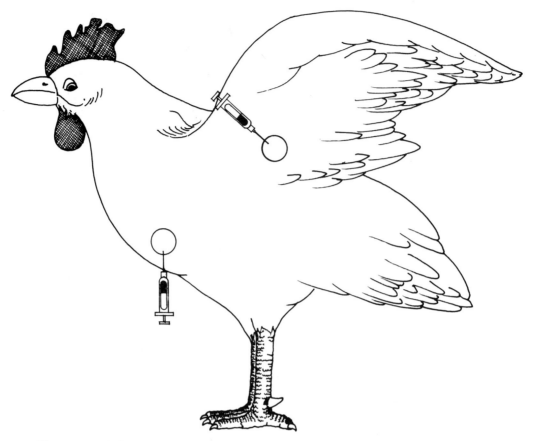

Figure 22.   Subcutaneous injection in poultry.

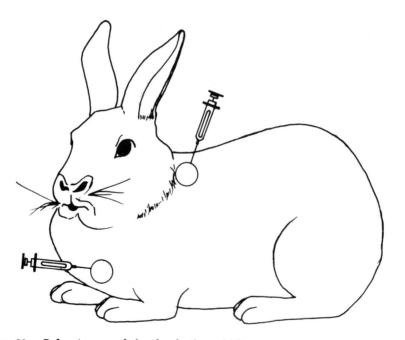

Figure 23.   Subcutaneous injection in the rabbit.

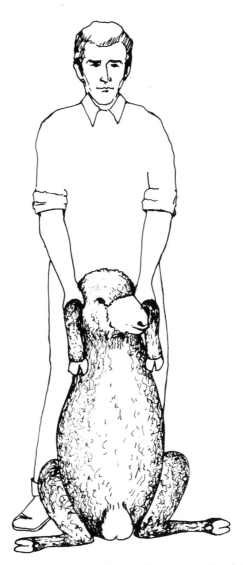

Figure 24. Restrain sheep and goats to give an intramuscular injection.

Intravenous

An intravenous injection is one that is made into a vein. It's used when the amount of solution that must be given is too large to be absorbed under the skin or when the product would irritate or harm the tissue.

The injection site in cattle, horses, mules, sheep, and goats is the left jugular vein. The jugulars are the large veins that carry blood from the head to the heart. They run from the back point of the jaw to the shoulder on each side of the neck.

The injection site in pigs is one of the veins on the outside of the ears; in birds an injection is made into a large vein found at the elbow on the inside of the wing.

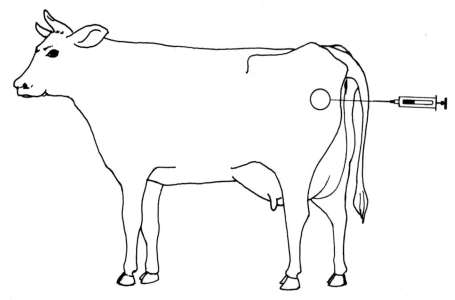

Figure 25.   Intramuscular injection in the cow.

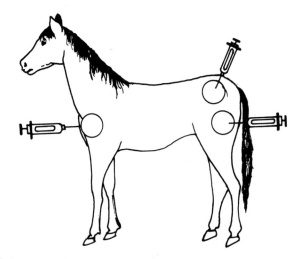

Figure 26.   Intramuscular injection in the horse and mule.

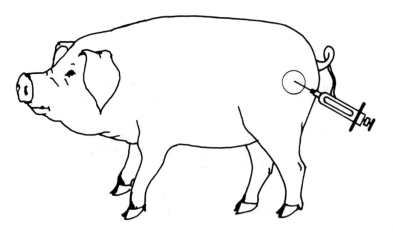

Figure 27a.   Intramuscular injection in the pig.

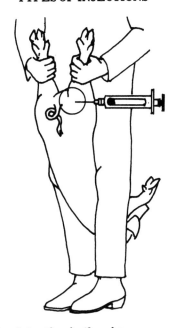

Figure 27b. Intramuscular injection in the pig.

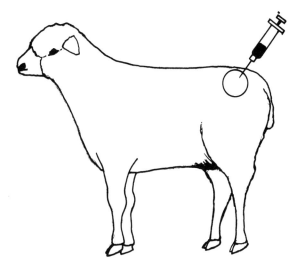

Figure 28. Intramuscular injection in sheep.

To make an intravenous injection the vein is compressed below the injection site in order to stop the flow of blood. The vein then enlarges making it easier to insert the needle.

In large animals it's convenient to use a rope tourniquet to stop the blood flow through the vein. The rope is placed around the neck of the animal, between the injection site and the animal's heart. As the rope is twisted tight with a stick, it squeezes a piece of cotton cloth or burlap material against the jugular. The vein engorges with blood and the needle is easily inserted. In smaller animals, such as pigs and birds, a helper or the person giving the injection should compress the vein using thumb pressure instead of a rope tourniquet.

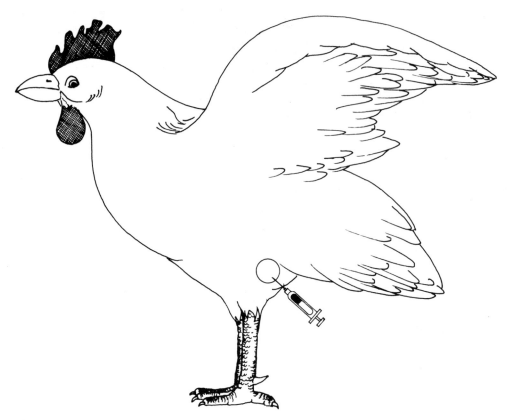

Figure 29.   Intramuscular injection in poultry.

Veins carry blood back toward the animal's heart. If air bubbles are accidentally introduced into a vein they will be carried along with the blood. This is very dangerous and could possibly kill the animal when they reach its heart! For this reason the needle is always inserted into the vein in the opposite direction to which the blood is flowing. The point of the needle must be inserted away from the heart (see Figure 30). If the insertion is done in this way there is less possibility of air entering the vein.

Before inserting the needle into the vein take it off its syringe or injection outfit. The needle should be held parallel to the vein with its bevel, the part of the tip with the hole in it, facing toward you. Insert the needle point through the skin in the same parallel direction. Pick up a little on the end of the needle that attaches to the syringe (causing the needle to become more vertical) and carefully push it through the wall of the vein.

When the needle point reaches the hollow center part of the vein lower the end of the needle back toward the vein and skin, causing it to become parallel once again. Now push the needle in its full length—making sure it's still in the center of the vein—to keep it from falling out.

If the insertion was done correctly you should see blood coming out of the open end of the needle. If no blood spurts from the open end it's possible that the bevel is pressed too tightly against the inside wall of the vein. If so, pull the needle out a little and rotate the needle point very slightly so that the bevel lies more in the center of the vein. Push the needle back in its full length.

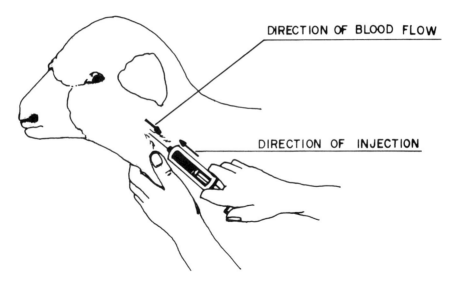

Figure 30.   Direction in which an intravenous injection is made.

Before attaching either a syringe, or the rubber or plastic tube of an injection outfit to the needle make sure they are full of the solution to be injected and no air bubbles remain inside. A good way to be sure there is no air inside either instrument is to let a few drops of the solution drip out before you attach the needle. After attaching the injection outfit you don't want the needle to move inside the vein while giving the shot. To keep this from happening tape the needle to the animal's skin with adhesive tape below the point where it connects to the injection outfit.

Once the syringe or injection outfit has been attached, and before making the injection, the pressure of the vein from the rope tourniquet or your thumb must be released. The rate at which the medicine is allowed to enter the vein must be very slow, especially when just beginning the injection. Large animals can receive 10–15 cubic centimeters (cc) the first minute; it should take at least 10 minutes to inject up to 300 cc. Smaller animals must receive smaller doses than these in the same time periods according to their weight and the manufacturer's instruction.

Usually a number 16 needle several inches long is used for cattle, horses, and mules. Smaller needles are used for smaller animals. To more strictly control the rate of flow of the medicine use a number 20 or a smaller needle. Depending on the species of the animal these very small needles will make it impossible to inject medicine too quickly.

If the flow of injected solution is too fast, the animal will go into shock—a condition in which the blood doesn't circulate through the body in the proper manner. It can be caused by hemorrhage, a serious infection, heart malfunction, or inability of the blood to absorb quickly enough large doses of powerful medicines. Signs that indicate shock are a rapid pulse, shortness of breath and quick breathing, a very rapid heart beat that may be irregular as well, frothing from the mouth (this looks like one of the symptoms of rabies), and collapse of the animal. Keep a close eye on any animal during an intravenous injection. If you do notice symptoms of shock stop the injection until the animal returns to its normal condition. When you resume, continue the injection at a slower rate of flow.

The figures I've given for the number of cubic centimeters that can be injected over a certain time period for large animals are general figures according to the type of animal. The same is true of the manufacturer's recommendations.

Each individual animal within the same breed has a slightly different body chemistry—as is the case with humans. Because of its body chemistry each animal will have a slightly different ability to absorb the same quantity of a medicine over the same length of time. Some will be able to absorb a little more, others a little less. As a result, one animal may go into shock when another one would have no difficulty absorbing the same dose. For this reason pay close attention to your animal during this type of injection. Using the manufacturer's recommended rate of flow as a maximum, reduce the speed of the flow according to each animal's ability to absorb the medicine (see Figures 31—cow; 32—horse; 33—pig; 34—fowl).

Intraperitoneal

Intraperitoneal injections are made in cattle with an injection outfit in order to administer large amounts of such solutions as calcium gluconate and dextrose. This type of injection is absorbed quickly, but not as fast as an intravenous one.

This is a dangerous injection and must be performed by someone with experience. The danger exists because the needle is inserted through the animal's skin, muscles, and peritoneum, and finally into the abdominal cavity—the part of the body that contains the stomach, intestines, and other organs. When penetrating this thin membrane you have to be absolutely certain the needle doesn't pierce any of the organs and that the solution is expelled into the hollow of the abdomen.

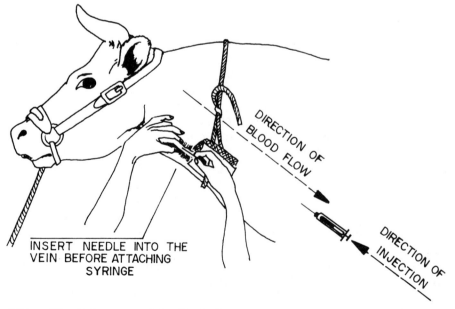

INSERT NEEDLE INTO THE VEIN BEFORE ATTACHING SYRINGE

DIRECTION OF BLOOD FLOW

DIRECTION OF INJECTION

Figure 31.   Intravenous injection in the cow.

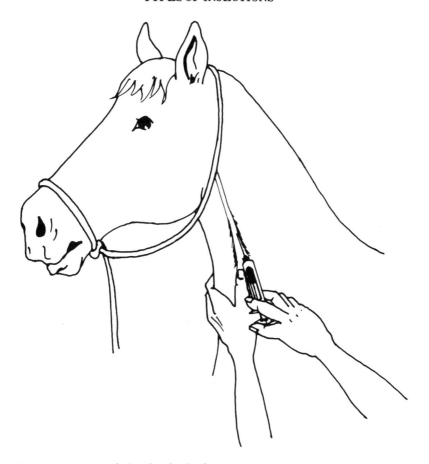

Figure 32.   Intravenous injection in the horse.

The needle is inserted into the center of the depression found in the animal's right side between the last rib and hipbone. Never use the cow's left side to make the injection or you may break through the rumen wall (the cow's first stomach).

Warm the solution or medicine to body temperature, but don't boil it. Then disinfect the injection site with alcohol or an iodine solution and put a long, sterilized needle on your syringe (a 2-inch number 16 or a 3-inch number 14). Finally, push the needle straight through the cow's skin, muscles, and peritoneum until it rests in the empty hollow of the abdominal cavity.

Make sure the needle has not penetrated an organ by moving it slightly from side to side. If the tip moves easily it's not in an organ. Connect the injection outfit and, using gravity, allow the solution to pass into the cow at the proper rate of flow.

Intrarumen

Intrarumen injections are occasionally made in cattle or sheep to treat the infection that commonly occurs when gas is released from the rumen and reticulum (the first and second stomachs of ruminant ani-

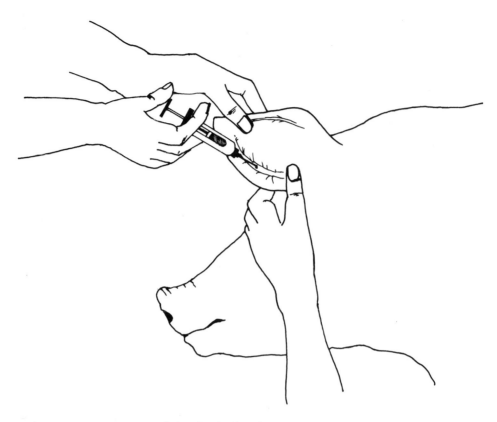

Figure 33.   Intravenous injection in the pig.

mals) when the rumen is punctured with a knife or trocar, a special instrument used to make a hole in the rumen, in a case of bloat (see Figure 35).

The injection site is always on the animal's left side in the center of an imaginary triangle drawn between the last rib, the hipbone, and the backbone. Use a 3-inch sterilized number 14 needle. To tell if the needle is in the right place draw it out slightly on the syringe plunger. This should fill the syringe with either gas or liquid escaping from the rumen (see Figure 36).

Intramammary

Intramammary infusions are used to treat an infected cow udder or teat, as in the case of bovine mastitis (see "Mastitis," p. 190 in Chapter 16, General Diseases of Domestic Animals).

Disinfect the teat and then squeeze it between your fingers as if you were milking. This will open the ring-shaped sphincter muscle that surrounds the teat opening and controls the release of milk. With the sphincter muscle open you can insert a sterilized canula, a small round-tipped tube with one or more holes in its sides (see Figure 37). Using either a syringe and needle, or a plastic injecting tube with medication already in it sold by the manufacturer, you can force medicine through the

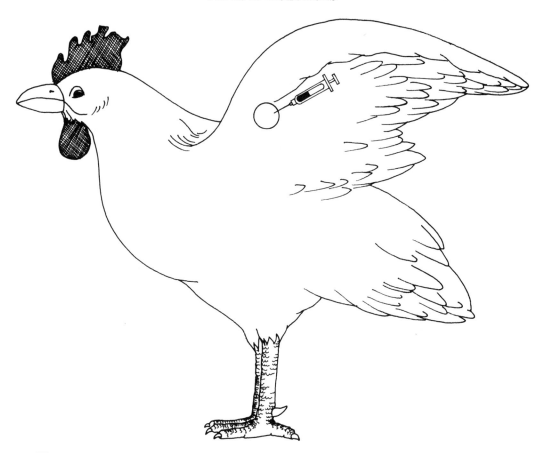

Figure 34.   Intravenous injection in poultry.

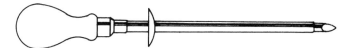

Figure 35.   A trocar used to relieve bloat in cattle.

canula and into the teat canal (the hollow space inside the teat where milk collects).

After giving the medicine 30 seconds to a minute to pass from the canula into the teat canal, remove the canula and disinfect the teat once again. The sphincter muscle will contract, closing the teat opening once the canula has been removed, and the medicine will be absorbed (see Figure 38).

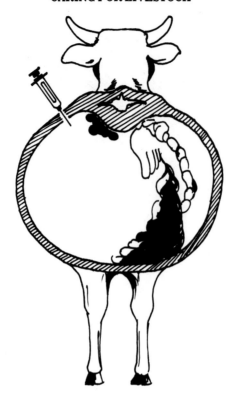

Figure 36.   Intrarumen injection in the cow.

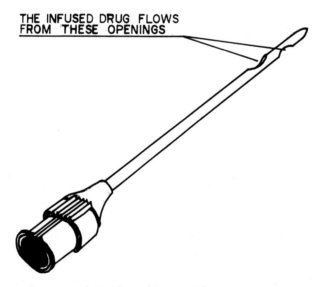

Figure 37.   Intramammary injection with a canula.

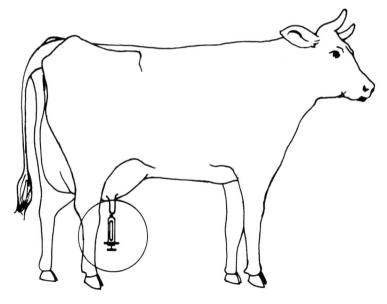

Figure 38.   Intramammary injection in the cow.

9

BIOLOGICAL PRODUCTS

Biological products are substances produced naturally within an animal's body or artificially in the laboratory. They are used to give immediate, temporary protection against attacking microorganisms and to cure the animal after such attacks, as in the case of immune blood serums, also called *antiserums* and *antitoxins,* or they may cause a longer lasting immunity, as with vaccines and bacterins. Other biological products called *diagnostics* and *diagnostic antigens* are used to detect and diagnose specific diseases.

Biological Products Can Diagnose Disease

Diagnostics and diagnostic antigens are made very much like bacterins. They are produced from living microbes that have been weakened or changed in structure in order to reduce their strength and ability to cause infection. Then they're killed.

Two common diagnostics are tuberculin, used as a test against tuberculosis, a bacterial disease that infects cattle, pigs, dogs, chickens, and people in its different forms, and mallein, used to test against glanders, a contagious bacterial disease that attacks horses, mules, burros, and people.

The tuberculosis test is conducted in the following manner: an intradermal injection of tuberculin is given to the test animal. If the animal has tuberculosis the injection site will swell and turn red within 1-3 days. The test for glanders is similar.

There are other kinds of diagnostic tests utilizing both in-the-field operations and laboratory techniques. These tests offer real advantages because they are so accurate in indicating disease—though they are never 100 percent effective—and do away with long quarantine periods. Before the discovery of *diagnostics,* quarantine and waiting for physical symptoms to appear were the only ways to deal with animals suspected of carrying disease.

Biological Products Need Help

Biological products are not able to do everything necessary to fight disease. They can cure animals of specific diseases, once they are infected, by imparting passive immunity, and can prevent the contraction of certain diseases over a long time period, by stimulating active immunity. But since they work within the animal's body they have no effect on its environment.

An animal's environment is the collection of conditions and influences that surround it and affect its development. Environment is usually one of the most important contributing factors to disease. For example, in warm climates pools of dirty water are perfect breeding grounds for all sorts of harmful microbes, mosquitoes, and other biting insects. If animals don't have access to a constant supply of clean drinking water, they will be forced to drink what's available, however dirty it is. And obviously, they will continually reinfect themselves with water-borne microorganisms.

Therefore, it is important to determine the contributing factors to each disease and eliminate them at the same time you treat infected and exposed animals with the biological products that are indicated. Do away with unsanitary conditions and provide proper housing and feed according to animal species.

Diseased animals are usually highly infectious. They produce enormous amounts of the harmful microbes associated with their illnesses. Depending on the particular disease these microorganisms are eliminated in urine, feces, nasal discharges, saliva, and other secretions. They can also be passed through common feed, water sources, and physical contact. Separate healthy animals from diseased ones and move them to disease-free areas.

The Use of Drugs, Medicines, and Biological Products

Drugs, medicines, and biological products come packaged with manufacturer's instructions that list the amount that should be injected according to an animal's weight and age. Read these instructions and follow them. They are the result of many years of research and testing and will serve as a useful guide.

If too little of an indicated substance is injected it may not cause enough or any of the desired effect in the animal. If too much is injected the animal may be injured, even to the point of death.

Most medicines and biological products are labeled with an expiration date, past which time the product will partially or completely lose its strength and effectiveness. Check this before buying anything.

Products left in the sun, direct light, or in warm places also lose their strength. It's important that they be stored in a cool and dark place. Nowadays, to protect against too much light exposure most medicine bottles are made of brown glass or plastic.

Biological products must be refrigerated but never frozen. They should be used as soon as possible after being removed from the refrigerator. If there is no electricity where you live, you don't have a refrigerator or access to one, or your animals are pastured far from the house, buy or build yourself a portable ice chest. An ice chest should serve to keep the vaccines cool for a day or two.

One thing to always remember is that certain kinds of vaccines are made from living agents (microbes). If you were to use chemical disinfectants on needles, syringes, injection outfits, and the injection site you would kill these agents and the vaccines would be of no use. Use lemon juice instead; it is a natural disinfectant and will not kill the living agents in the vaccine.

Biological products have to be shaken well before being injected so that the active agent is mixed evenly throughout the product. Destroy unused supplies and empty bottles according to the manufacturer's recommendations so as to not spread disease.

Vaccination Checklist

1. Maintain a regular preventive vaccination schedule against the diseases to which your animals are susceptible. Prevention is cheap, it's the cure that's expensive! Vaccinate at the proper point in your animal's life.
2. If an animal becomes infected, identify the specific disease. Also, you must assume its herdmates have been exposed as well.
3. Only buy biological products from reputable veterinary supply houses that keep their biologicals refrigerated.
4. Check to see that the expiration date is far enough in the future so that you'll be able to use the product knowing that it will have the required potency.
5. Make sure the metal seal of the bottle top has not been opened or tampered with.
6. Carry biologicals out of the sun and keep them refrigerated (in your own ice chest, if need be).
7. Store vaccines in a refrigerator or ice chest. Never let them freeze.
8. Sterilize syringes and needles by boiling at least 10 minutes.
9. Never use a chemical disinfectant on injection equipment when injecting attenuated or live vaccines. (Attenuated vaccines are made in the laboratory from living microorganisms that have been weakened.) Chemical disinfectants will kill the living agents in the vaccines causing them to become worthless.
10. It's all right to use chemical disinfectants on injection equipment when injecting inactivated vaccines (those that contain microorganisms that have been killed and are able to multiply), antiserums (immune blood serums), and toxoids (toxins that have changed so they're no longer poisonous but can still stimulate the production of antitoxins).

11. Disinfect the rubber stopper of any bottle containing a biological product (except live vaccines) with a piece of sterile cotton dipped in alcohol before passing a needle through it. Live vaccine rubber bottle tops are to be disinfected with lemon juice.
12. Shake the bottle of vaccine to distribute the active agents throughout the mixture.
13. Use a sterile needle for removing any product from its bottle and disinfect it with alcohol before each injection, except when injecting live vaccines.
14. Properly dispose of unused vaccines and the containers they came in according to the manufacturer's instructions.
15. Keep the following records:
    a. vaccine name and manufacturer
    b. the name of the veterinary supply house from which you bought the vaccine
    c. the vaccine's serial number
    d. expiration date
    e. the number of vaccinated animals and some way of identifying them
    f. the date the vaccination was given
    g. the dosage injected
    h. any reactions observed after the vaccination.

These records are important for a number of reasons: to build a vaccination history of each of your animals which will influence their sale prices, to know when to vaccinate next, and whether your animals are already protected if a particular disease breaks out.

10

THREE CLASSES OF VETERINARY DRUGS

Sulfonamides, also called *sulfa drugs* and *nitrofurans* (both of which are man-made chemicals), and antibiotics (formed by fungi, molds, and bacteria) are three different types of powerful agents used to treat disease. They work in two ways, depending on the specific infection: by killing the attacking microorganisms or by interfering with their growth or reproduction. This interference with a microbe's normal life processes allows an animal's natural defenses to overwhelm and destroy the invader.

Some of the drugs within each of these main classes are selective in the way they act. They only affect one particular harmful microorganism. Others are called broad spectrum drugs; they work against many different kinds of microorganisms. Each type is useful. A selective drug, also called a *specific drug* is used when one attacking organism can be clearly identified as being the cause of disease. A broad spectrum drug should be given when a disease may be caused by several closely related organisms or several unrelated microbes on which it has an inhibiting or deadly effect.

Many diseases are caused by a number of harmful germs. Mastitis, an inflammation of the udder, can be caused by bacteria, molds, yeasts, viruses, and also mechanical injury. More than two dozen pathogenic microbes are also able to produce mastitis. This is the sort of disease that must be treated with a broad spectrum drug.

A drug used to treat a disease in one species of animal may not have any effect on the same disease in another kind of animal, and, if by chance it does, the dosage will almost certainly be different. In the same way, a drug that cures one particular disease may or may not cure others, no matter how closely related they may be.

Some disease germs develop resistance to particular drugs and are not affected by their use. Resistance is related to how frequently and at what dosage drugs are given. In particular, bacteria sometimes become resistant to an antibiotic that previously would kill them, especially if the drug was first given at too low a dosage. Resistance is most often developed against the antibiotic streptomycin. Once a microorganism develops resistance against a certain antibiotic other antibiotics with nearly the same structure or same way of fighting the germ usually have no effect on it either.

Prevent Drug Resistance

1. Don't use drugs carelessly; follow the manufacturer's directions.
2. In general, don't apply drugs to only one part of the animal's body (locally); make sure they're given in the proper manner.
3. Give the correct dosage according to animal species, age, body weight, and level of seriousness of the disease (again following the manufacturer's instructions).
4. Only use drugs in combination when they've been tested and proven effective.
5. Change drugs when you notice the first signs of resistance.

The Ideal Drug

The ideal drug:

1. works against many different kinds of microorganisms (has a broad spectrum effect);
2. is not poisonous to the animal being treated;
3. has a very small tendency to produce resistance in the attacking microorganism;
4. doesn't harm or kill the beneficial organisms that normally live within an animal's system.

Sulfonamides (Sulfa Drugs)

Sulfonamides limit the growth and reproduction of harmful bacteria, letting the animal's defenses overwhelm the disease-causing infection. In general they are effective against a wide range of pathogenic bacteria and are helpful in treating secondary bacterial invasions. Sulfa drugs are of no use against viruses.

Once the first symptoms of bacterial infection are recognized sulfonamides must be used quickly, but in long-lasting diseases the sulfa drugs are ineffective. This is because chronic infections weaken body defenses to the point where they can't kill harmful bacteria that have been kept from multiplying by the sulfonamides. If by chance these drugs are used to treat a long-term infection the disease-causing germs become more resistant to future treatment.

Since most of the sulfonamides have a similar structure, once a microorganism shows signs that it's resistant to one drug in the group it is probably resistant to others. Resistance is usually produced from too low a dosage.

When using sulfa drugs it is important to keep a constant level in all parts of the animal's body where the harmful microorganisms might spread. Therefore, it's best to give the drugs orally as tablets at regular intervals during a 24-hour period or in powdered form mixed into the feed. The average dosage is 1-½ grains (15 grains = 1 gram) per pound of animal body weight, but check the manufacturer's recommendations for exact amounts.

A good rule of thumb is that if a positive reaction is not shown to sulfonamide use within 3 days the drug should be discontinued. If a positive reaction is shown the dosage should be lowered. Treatment may continue up to 6 days, but no longer. Once an animal appears healthy again, it should continue to be given the required sulfa drug for another 1-½ days, up to the maximum of 6 days for the total treatment. This is in order to prevent a relapse (the return of the disease condition).

The prolonged use of sulfonamides may cause toxic (poisonous) reactions in different animals. A few of the signs are diarrhea, constipation, anemia, loss of appetite, skin rash, excitement or depression, and other reactions. Chickens may lay fewer eggs. The most common signs of toxicity are frequent and bloody urination. Stop treatment immediately if such conditions appear.

The biggest problem with the sulfa drugs is that they don't dissolve easily in body fluids. If given in too high a dosage or for too long a time they tend to collect in the kidneys. When the concentration of the drug becomes high enough it crystallizes (changes to its solid form) in the shape

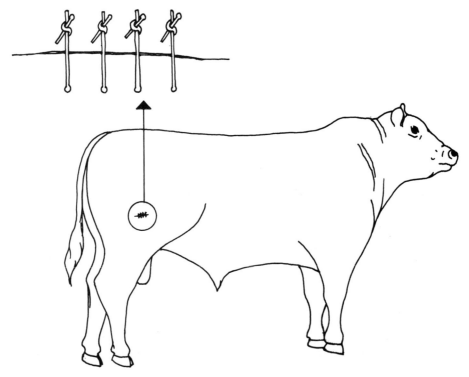

Figure 39.   Apply 50 mg of a sulfa drug per square inch to sutured wounds.

of little needles. These needles cut and tear the inner lining of the kidneys and may in time form stones that block body wastes from being excreted. If this continues to happen the animal will ultimately die. When treating a disease condition with sulfonamides always let the animal have constant access to clean, fresh water.

Sulfonamides are most commonly given orally. When it's not possible to do that or it's necessary to quickly raise their level in the blood, they can be administered via an intravenous or intraperitoneal injection. Sulfa drugs are also used (as a sterile powder) for local wounds, but they must first be cleaned. Apply 50 milligrams per square inch to sutured wounds (see Figure 39). Use 100 milligrams per square inch on open and very contaminated wounds.

Nitrofurans

Nitrofurans are man-made chemicals produced from peanut shells, oat hulls, corn cobs, and beet pulp, and they are used to kill many kinds of bacteria. If they're used for a long time they may upset the animal's stomach and intestines, reduce normal weight gains, or decrease sperm production in the male.

Depending on the type of infection an animal has it is important to use the nitrofuran that is specifically indicated.

Antibiotics

Antibiotics are naturally produced antibacterial chemicals that interfere with the growth of infectious germs. In large dosages they kill harmful bacteria; in lower concentrations they limit bacterial growth.

Most antibiotics are selective in their action and only useful against certain specific kinds of bacterial infections. Others, the broad spectrum antibiotics, can be used against many kinds of bacterial diseases.

Antibiotics are usually given by intramuscular injection, and less often, when necessary intravenously. If they are given orally they interfere with the function of beneficial bacteria in the digestive tract.

If no change for the better is seen in an infected animal's condition while being treated with a specific or broad spectrum antibiotic during a 48-hour period, it is time to change drugs. Either try another antibiotic or a different class of antibacterial drug.

Some bacteria will develop resistance to an antibiotic that previously killed them, especially if the antibiotic was originally used in too low a dosage. Antibiotics produce less toxic effects than sulfonamides but you must watch out for allergic reactions. If an animal shows signs of allergy to a particular antibiotic stop treatment immediately.

If the skin, ear, eye, udder, or other localized spot on the animal's body is infected it's possible to use an antibiotic on just that one spot. However, if a local infection is very bad it's best to use two antibiotics—one on the particular spot and the other injected, in order to treat the animal's whole body (known as a systemic treatment).

In the case of bovine mastitis, intramammary injections of antibiotics are given. These antibiotics then appear in the milk for a certain time afterward. During this time none of the affected milk products should be used for human consumption, although they can be fed to animals. Pay close attention to the manufacturer's recommendations about the use of milk products while a cow is receiving or just after it receives an antibiotic treatment.

11

DRUG GUIDE

This guide is divided into five columns: Drug Class, Chemical Name (with the common name in parentheses below it), Diseases, Dosage, and Other Information.

Drug Class tells which of the three general classes of veterinary drugs the medicine belongs to— sulfonamides (sulfa drugs), antibiotics, or nitrofurans. The chemical name is the name by which a drug is officially known based on its chemical composition. The common name is the name it may more popularly be known by. The Diseases column lists by animal species the diseases each drug is used against for either prevention or treatment. The final classification, Other Information, lists by disease the toxic reactions caused by a medicine, the specific form of the drug that should be used, what other drugs can replace it, and other important information.

The example below will best illustrate how to make use of the Drug Guide.

Drug Class	Chemical Name (common name)	Disease	Dosage	Other Information
Antibiotic	Oxytetracycline (terramycin)	1. *Horses:* a. Anthrax	*Horses a.* Early in the disease give a first injection (IV) of 2 gm, then every 12 hrs 1.5 gm (IV)	*Horses a.* Penicillin can be used instead, early in the disease. Give (IM) 6 million units of procaine penicillin G (in aqueous solution)

In our example read left to right. The Drug Class is antibiotic; the chemical name of this particular drug is oxytetracycline, but it is more commonly known as terramycin. One of the diseases it is used to treat in horses is anthrax, a very deadly infection caused by a bacilli bacteria (see Chapter 2, Bacteria and Viruses) and its spore form. As you continue reading to the right you'll see that the dosage of terramycin that's injected intravenously (IV) early in the disease is 2 grams. Then every 12 hours afterward an additional intravenous injection (IV) of 1.5 gm. is given. After reading Chapter 8, Types of Injections, you know how and where to give an intravenous injection to a horse.

The last column, Other Information, tells you that penicillin, another medicine from the same drug class, can be substituted for terramycin. This is important to know in case you can't find a supply of terramycin. Penicillin is measured in units rather than grams or milligrams. The instructions call for an intramuscular injection (IM) of procaine penicillin G, a specific form of the drug, in an aqueous solution. This means the drug comes premixed in its bottle in a solution of serile water.

Abbreviations Used

IM	intramuscular
IV	intravenous
IMM	intramammary
SC	subcutaneous
gm	grams
mg	milligrams
mg/lb body wt	milligrams per pound of body weight
qts	quarts
gal	gallon
hrs	hours
lb	pound
ml	milliliter

A Partial Listing of Terms Used

Any unfamiliar terms used in the drug guide that are not explained here will be found in the glossary at the end of the book.

acute	severe
aqueous	containing water
atrophic	wasting away
cecal	the beginning of the large intestine
enteric	of the intestines
hemorrhagic	to have heavy bleeding
hepatic	of the liver
infusion	the slow introduction of a solution into a part of the body
itis	a word ending, meaning inflammation of a part of the body
locally	a particular part of the body
necrotic	death or decay causing (in the tissue of a specific part of the body)
solution	when one or more liquids, gases, or solids are mixed together so as to dissolve or merge completely
suspension	when a substance is dispersed through a liquid but not dissolved in it

A Warning about Drug Use

Drugs are very powerful tools in the fight to prevent and treat disease. However, they must be prescribed properly, administered in the indicated dosage, and given in the correct manner at the right time. Most of all, they can't be thought of and used as miracle workers. They have their place in management practice but cannot be used to obscure faults in other important areas such as nutrition, housing, and preventative health care.

In the following drug guide several drugs are mentioned as possible treatments for the same disease. Quite often there is one that gives more effective results than others, and if so, it is pointed out.

The beginning point for any farmer, after noticing the first disease symptoms in an animal, is diagnosis, finding out what has made it sick. Diagnosis is usually difficult, but we have to do the best we can. When there is time it's a very good idea to take a specimen (blood, saliva, urine, milk, feces, a piece of an organ when an animal has died, and so forth) from the animal and send it to a professional laboratory for analysis. (The specimen you take will depend on the nature of the disease.) In this way you have a better chance of correctly identifying the disease and then deciding what action to take, be it drug application or some other management practice. Never hesitate to call in a veterinarian when you are in doubt, or to utilize the extension and laboratory services of your state agricultural university. By all means learn and profit from your practical experience.

Class of Drug	Chemical Name (Common Name)	Disease	Dosage	Other Information
Sulfonamide (sulfa drugs)	Sulfamerazine	1. *Horse, Mule:* a. Pneumonia b. Strangles (equine distemper) c. Fistulous withers (inflammation of the back between the shoulder blades) d. Poll evil (inflammation of top or back of the head) e. Some intestinal diseases in foals f. Some blood diseases in foals 2. Cattle: a. Acute mastitis with blood poisoning b. Calf pneumonia c. Foot rot d. Calf diphtheria	*For All Farm Animals Except Poultry:* *Orally:* 60 mg/lb body wt. The dosage should be divided in half and given twice a day. (Every 12 hrs give 30 mg/lb body wt) *Intravenous Injection:* Only give (IV) injections using sodium sulfamerazine. The dose is 30 mg/lb body wt once a day *For Poultry (not for any other type of animal):* Sodium sulfamerazine can be mixed into drinking water at a ratio of 1–2 measures of sodium sulfamerazine to 1000 measures of water. This means you mix 1–2 teaspoons of sodium sulfamerazine to every 5 quarts of water used for drinking *Cattle c.:* 30–60 mg sodium sulfamerazine / lb body wt given (IV) daily for 4 days	*Cattle a.* Sulfamerazine should be used with an antibiotic. (IMM) and (IM) injections are given at the same time *Cattle b.* Sulfamethazine can be used instead *Cattle c.* Use sodium sulfamerazine *Cattle d.* Treatment must be given as rapidly as possible after noticing disease symptoms. Sulfamethazine and sulfapyridine may also be used. Or penicillin, either alone or in combination with sulfamerazine, sulfamethazine, or sulfapyridine

Disease	Dosage	Notes
e. Calf scours		
f. Metritis (inflammation of the uterus)		
3. *Pigs:*		*Pigs a.* Sulfamerazine can be used alone or together with sulfamethazine
a. Pneumonia		
4. *Poultry:*		*Poultry a., b., c.* Sulfamerazine will reduce the number of birds that die from these 3 diseases
a. Pullorum disease		
b. Fowl typhoid		*Poultry c.* Sodium sulfamerazine (may be toxic) is given in the feed 5–7 days, or use sulfamethazine in the feed or drinking water
c. Infectious coryza		
Sulfamethazine (Sulfadimidine)	For All Animals Except Poultry: *Orally:* 22.5 mg/lb body wt every 12 hrs *(IV) Injection:* 30 mg/lb body wt once daily	*All Species:* (IV) Injection of sulfamethazine must be done slowly to prevent severe shock
1. *Horses, Mules:*		
a. Pneumonia		
b. Strangles		
c. Fistulous withers	For Poultry (not for other kinds of animals): Sulfamethazine can be mixed into feed at the ratio of 1 part sulfamethazine to 200 parts feed. For example, in 1 kg of feed you would mix 5 mg of sulfamethazine. Sodium sulfamethazine should be mixed into drinking water at a ratio of between 1 and 2 teaspoons per 5 quarts of water	
d. Navel ill of foals		*Horses d.* Streptomycin alone or with penicillin may also be used.
2. *Cattle:*		*Cattle a.* Sulfamethazine may be used alone or with antibiotics, given (IMM) and (IM) at the same time
a. Acute mastitis with blood poisoning		
b. Calf pneumonia		*Cattle b.* Sulfamerazine can be used instead

Class of Drug	Chemical Name (Common Name)	Disease	Dosage	Other Information
		c. Calf diphtheria d. Calf metritis e. Calf scours (Infectious diarrhea)		*Cattle c.* Treatment must be given as soon as possible after disease symptoms appear. Sulfamerazine and sulfapyridine may also be used or penicillin, either alone or in combination with sulfamethazine, sulfamerazine, or sulfapyridine
		f. Foot rot	*Cattle f.* Give 30 mg/lb body wt (IV) daily for 4 days	*Cattle f.* Use sodium sulfamethazine
		g. Pneumonic pasteurellosis (shipping fever)	*Cattle g.* First give 60 mg/lb body wt orally or by (IV) injection. Follow this with 30 mg/lb body wt given orally every 12 hrs for 3–4 days. Or, give 30 mg/lb body wt of sodium sulfamethazine by (IV) injection once daily for 4 days	*Cattle g.* Dihydrostreptomycin with penicillin can be used (when the disease has just started). Oxytetracycline also works well. No matter what drug is used treatment must be started as soon as the first signs of disease are noticed
		3. *Sheep:* a. Certain kinds of mastitis (caused by Pasteurella) b. Certain kinds of pneumonia (caused by Pasteurella)		
		4. *Rabbits:* a. Intestinal coccidiosis b. Hepatic coccidiosis		*Rabbits a.* Used for treatment of the disease *Rabbits b.* Used in prevention and treatment
		5. *Poultry:* a. Pullorum disease b. Fowl typhoid		*Poultry a.* Used for treatment of the disease *Poultry b.* Used in prevention and treatment

Drug	Diseases	Dosage	Notes
	c. Fowl cholera d. Paratyphoid e. Infectious coryza 6. *Pigs:* a. Rhinitis (bull-nose, sniffles)	*Pigs a.* First give 60 mg/lb body wt orally or (IV). Follow this with 30 mg/lb body wt every 12 hours during 3–4 days. If you use sodium sulfamethazine give an (IV) injection of 30 mg/lb body wt daily for 4 days	*Poultry a–e.* Sulfamethazine will reduce the numbers of birds that die from these diseases

Sulfanilamide	1. *Horses, Mules:*
	   a. Pneumonia
	   b. Bronchitis
	   c. Strangles
	   d. Infected wounds (generally)
		Horses and Mules: 30 mg/lb body wt given every 12 hours	*Horses c.* Penicillin, sulfamerazine and sulfamethazine may also be used
			 Horses d. Applied locally to the wound itself or given orally

Sulfathiazole	1. *Cattle:*
	   a. Urinary Infections
	   b. Foot rot
	 2. *Pigs:*
	   a. Infect. enteritis (pig typhoid)
	   b. Pneumonia
	   c. Pasteurellosis (swine plague)
	   d. Oily skin
	 3. *Poultry:*
	   a. Fowl cholera
	   b. Infectious coryza (in chickens)
		Cattle and Pigs: 120–180 mg/lb body wt given daily orally (in total). Divide total dose into equal parts to be given every 4–6 hours. If you treat the animal every 4 hrs. give 20–30 mg/lb body wt. If treatment is made every 6 hrs. give 30–45 mg/lb body wt	*Cattle b.* Use Sodium sulfathiazole
			 Pigs a. A combination of streptomycin (IM) and streptomycin or nitrofurazone orally can also be used
			 Pigs d. A 3% sulfathiazole ointment is used locally
			 Poultry a. and b. Sulfathiazole reduces the number of deaths from these 2 diseases

Class of Drug	Chemical Name (Common Name)	Disease	Dosage	Other Information

	Sulfaquinoxaline	1. *Cattle:*
		  a. Intestinal cocci-diosis (in calves)
		2. *Sheep:*
		  a. Intestinal cocci-diosis (of lambs)
		3. *Poultry:*
		  a. Coccidiosis
		
		  b. Acute fowl cholera
		
		  c. Fowl typhoid
		
		4. *Rabbits:*
		  a. Hepatic coc-cidiosis
		
		  b. Intestinal cocci-diosis
			Follow manufacturer's directions carefully as dosages vary according to the manner in which the drug is given and whether it is used for prevention or treatment
			
			Rabbits a. for rabbits heavily exposed to this disease give 1/4 tsp mixed in 5 qts drinking water constantly during 30 days. For prevention use the treatment given for Rabbits b
			Rabbits b. For treatment mix 1 gm with each kg of feed given during 2 weeks
				Poultry: a. Used to treat coccidiosis in chickens and to both prevent and treat it in turkeys
				Poultry b. When added to the feed reduces the number of chickens that will die from the disease
				Poultry c. Add the drug to the drinking water to reduce the number of deaths in turkeys
				
				Rabbits a. and b. Use sodium sulfaquinoxaline. Do not feed the drug within 10 days of slaughter

	Sulfisoxazole	1. *Cattle:*
		  a. Urinary tract infections
		  b. Foot rot
		  c. Pasteurellosis (shipping fever)
		  d. Pneumonia
		  e. Mastitis
			Cattle:
			General dosage is 15–22.5 mg/lb body wt every 5 hours
				Cattle e. Given as an (IMM) injection

	Drug	Indications	Dosage	Notes
	Succinylsulfa-thiazole (sulfathialidine)	1. *Cattle:* a. Calf Scours 2. *Pigs:* a. Infectious enteritis (pig typhoid)	*Cattle and Pigs:* 60–135 mg/lb body wt given orally once daily	
	Homosulfanilamide Hydrochloride (sulfamylon)	1. *In All Animal Species* a. Infected wounds 2. *Cattle:* a. Metritis		*All Animal Species a.* Use a powder on the wound that contains 1 part homosulfanilamide to 8 parts sulfanilamide *Cattle a.* A suspension containing both homosulfanilamide and sulfanilamide is introduced into the uterus
	Phthalylsulface-tamide	1. *Young Animals Of All Species:* a. Intestinal infections	*Young Animals of All Species:* 13–40 mg/lb body wt given orally every 8 hrs	*Young Animals:* Phthalylsulfacetamide is used in many medicines that treat diarrhea
Antibiotics	Penicillin	1. *Horses, Mules:* a. Strangles 2. *Cattle:* a. Some kinds of mastitis b. Infectious cystitis (inflammation of the urinary tract)	*Horses a.* In combination give (IM) or (IV) 3,000–10,000 units of penicillin G potassium or sodium/lb body wt and (IM) the same dose as above of procaine penicillin in an aqueous solution. Repeat this second injection every 24 hrs *Cattle b.* Treatment must be started as soon as disease symptoms are shown. Give 3,000–10,000 units of procaine penicillin G in a sterile water suspension/lb body wt once a day during 8–15 days	*Horses a.* Treatment must be started before abscesses are formed. Once it's started it must be continued until the temperature drops to normal and for a few days afterward *Cattle a.* Generally used in combination with strep-tomycin, terramycin, or aureomycin. Given by (IMM) injection

Class of Drug	Chemical Name (Common Name)	Disease	Dosage	Other Information
		c. Metritis		Cattle c. A suspension of penicillin is introduced into the uterus
		d. Anthrax	Cattle d. Mature cattle receive up to 6 million units daily	Catle d. Only sick animals receive penicillin treatment; healthy ones are vaccinated Disease must be treated as soon as symptoms appear
		e. Foot rot	Cattle e. 3,000–10,000 units of procaine penicillin G in aqueous solution/lb body wt given (IM) once a day	Cattle e. One injection given early in the disease will usually cure it
		f. Calf pneumonia		
		3. Poultry: a. Erysipelas	Poultry a. All infected birds get 5,000 units/lb body wt of procaine penicillin by (SC) or (IM) injection and must get an injection of E. Insidiosa bacterin simultaneously	Poultry a. Streptomycin (injected) or oxytetracycline (given orally) can be substituted for penicillin
		4. In All Animal Species: a. Infections of the skin, ears, and eyes	All Animal Species a. Depending on the infection and how serious it is a minimum dose of 2,000 units per lb body wt is given (IM). In serious infections the dose is raised to 5,000–10,000 units/lb body wt. Frequency of treatment depends on how the drug is prepared: in aqueous solution every 3–4 hrs; in oil and beeswax every 12 hrs; when the drug is meant to act over a long period every 24 hrs or longer	All Animal Species a. A penicillin ointment is applied locally. In severe infections an (IM) injection is given as well
	Streptomycin and Dihydrostreptomicyn	1. Horses, Mules: a. Blood poisoning of new born foals	Horses a. Foals are given 0.5 gm (IM) every 3–4 hrs	Horses a. A combination of streptomycin and penicillin is usually best for this condition

Disease	Treatment	Notes
2. *Cattle:*		
a. Mastitis	*Cattle a.* Try an (IMM) injection of 0.5 gm twice a day. If no reaction, give 5 gm (IMM) and 5–7 gm (IM) twice a day	*Cattle a.* Used usually with penicillin as a combined (IMM) injection
b. Calf pneumonia		*Cattle b.* Continue treatment 4–5 days
c. Vibriosis	*Cattle c.* For cows infuse a mixture of 1 gm streptomycin and 10 ml distilled water into the uterus. For bulls give 25 gm (IM) and a mixture of 5 gm streptomycin in 10 ml of sterile salt water put into the sheath of the penis and massaged around the penis 5 minutes a day for 3 days	*Cattle c.* Can also be mixed with penicillin for the uterine infusion
d. Metritis		*Cattle d.* Combined with penicillin for a uterine infusion
3. *Pigs:*		
a. Leptospirosis	*Pigs a.* 5–10 mg/pound body wt given (IM) every 12 hours for 3 days.	
4. *Poultry:*		
a. Infectious sinusitis in turkeys		*Poultry a.* Injected into the turkey's sinus region. Tylosin is the most effective drug for this disease. If the turkey is very sick streptomycin may kill it
b. Chronic respiratory disease of chickens		*Poultry b.* Injected locally; followed by 3–4 days of mixing the drug in the drinking water. Tylosin is more effective. Secondary bacterial invaders must also be treated for

Class of Drug	Chemical Name (Common Name)	Disease	Dosage	Other Information
		5. *All Animal Species:* a. Intestinal infections	General Dosage: *Horses:* 1–2 mg/lb body wt (IM) every 3 to 4 hrs *Calves and Pigs.* For intestinal infections 1 gm orally once a day *Poultry.* 15–50 mg/lb body wt when injected *Small animals.* 10 mg/lb body wt (IM) or (SC) injection given every 12 hours. 5 mg/lb body wt if given every 6 hrs	*All Animal Species a.* Generally should be helpful. Given orally *Toxic Reactions:* Occur when large doses are given over long time periods. Streptomycin infrequently causes permanent hearing loss; dihydrostreptomycin causes it more often and should only be used if no other drug gives results. Persons handling streptomycin may get dermatitis
	Tetracycline (Achromycin)	1. *Horses, Mules:* a. Strangles	*Large Animals:* *Orally.* 2.5–5 mg/lb body wt *(IM) or (IV) Injection* every 12 hrs. 2–5 mg/lb body wt daily	*Horses a.* Penicillin is the preferred drug
		2. *Cattle:* a. Foot rot	*Small Animals:* *Orally.* 12.5–25 mg/lb body wt every 12 hrs *(IM) or (IV) Injection.* 2.5 mg/lb body wt every 12 hrs	*Cattle a.* Penicillin is usually given or else sulfamerazine or sulfamethazine
		b. Calf scours		*Cattle b.* Tetracycline is used to treat secondary bacterial invaders
		3. *All Species:* a. Infected wounds	*All Species:* *Orally.* First give 10–25 mg/lb body wt of chlortetracycline hydrochloride. Then every 12 hrs afterward give 5–12.5 mg/lb body wt *(IV) Injection.* A first dose of 2–5 mg/lb body wt. Then, every 12 hrs	*Toxic Reactions:* (IM) injections sometimes cause pain and inflame the injection site. Oral application in adult cows, sheep, and goats will kill normal bacteria found in the rumen

| Chlortetracycline (Aureomycin) | 1. *Horses, Mules:*
  a. Strangles
  b. Shipping fever
  c. Pneumonia
  d. Blood poisoning of newborn foals
2. *Cattle:*
  a. Metritis
  b. Foot rot
  c. Shipping fever
  d. Pneumonia
  e. Calf scours
  f. Listeriosis (Circling disease)

  g. Anaplasmosis | afterward give 1–2.5 mg/lb body wt. The injection must be given slowly with a 2.5% solution of the drug

Cattle f.
Orally: 15–50 mg/lb body wt daily (in total). Should be divided into 2 or more equal doses
(IV) Injection: 1–2.5 mg/lb body wt every 12 hrs. Continue treatment 24 hrs after body temperature has returned to normal
Cattle g.
Prevention. 0.5 mg/lb body wt daily given in the feed up to 60 days
Treatment of Infection. 5 mg/lb body wt injected daily for 10 days in a row | *Horses a.* Penicillin is generally used
Horses b. Must be used 3–4 days

Cattle b. Penicillin is usually given

Cattle f. To be given in the highest dosage the animal can tolerate; in spite of this it may die |

Class of Drug	Chemical Name (Common Name)	Disease	Dosage	Other Information
		3. *Pigs:* a. Infect. Necrotic enteritis (pig typhoid)		*Pigs a.* A combination of streptomycin (IM) and streptomycin or nitrofurazone orally can also be given. None of these drugs, including Aureomycin, is completely effective
		b. Swine dysentery (bloody scours)		*Pigs b.* Tylosin is the most commonly used antibacterial
		c. Salmonellosis (paratyphoid)		*Pigs c.* Nitrofurazone is also used for the intestinal form of the disease (given orally)
		4. *Poultry:* a. Infect. Synovitis (infect. arthritis)	*Poultry a.* The best treatment is 100 mg of Aureomycin added to 1 lb of feed	*Poultry a.* Oxytetracycline in the feed or an (IM) injection of 200 mg of streptomycin, early in the disease can also be used.
		b. Fowl typhoid		*Poultry b.* Aureomycin reduces the number of deaths from the disease but the best treatment is 100 mg of furazolidone in each lb of feed
		c. Blue Comb disease of chickens	*Poultry c.* Mix 1 gm Aureomycin in each gal of water for a week; then, stop water treatment and feed 100–200 mg of the same drug mixed into each lb of feed for 2 weeks	

Drug	Disease	Dosage	Notes
Oxytetracycline (terramycin)	1. *Horses, Mules:* a. Anthrax	*Horses a.* Early in the disease give a first injection of 2 gm (IV), then every 12 hrs 1.5 gm (IV)	*Horses a.* Penicillin can be used instead. Early in the disease give 6 million units of procaine penicillin G in aqueous suspension (IM)
	b. Strangles		*Horses b.* Penicillin is more commonly used
	c. Pneumonia d. Fistulous withers	*Horses d.* 3–5 mg/lb body wt daily given (IM) or (IV). Or 15–16.5 mg/lb body wt is given orally every 8 hours	*Horses d.* Terramycin may also be used locally on the infected spot
	2. *Cattle:* a. Mastitis	*Cattle a.* In very acute attacks give 3–5 mg/lb body wt (IM) or (IV) daily. At the same time give an (IMM) injection once daily. Treatment should be continued 3–4 days	*Cattle a.* Usually given by (IMM) injection
	b. Shipping fever	*Cattle b.* 5–10 mg/lb body wt (IM) or (IV) once a day for 3 days	*Cattle b.* When recognized early give a combined injection of dihydrostreptomycin and penicillin. Sulfamethazine can be used instead. Whichever drug or drug combination is used, continue treatment 3–4 days
	c. Metritis		
	d. Foot rot		*Cattle d.* Penicillin, sulfamerazine, or sulfamethazine are usually used early in the disease
	e. Anthrax	*Cattle e.* Same dosage as for horses	
	f. Calf scours	*Cattle f.* A generalized infection is treated with an (IM) or (IV) injection of 3 mg/lb body wt daily	

Class of Drug	Chemical Name (Common Name)	Disease	Dosage	Other Information
		3. *Sheep:* a. Diarrhea		*Sheep.* Given in the feed
		4. *Pigs:* a. Necrotic enteritis (pig typhoid)		*Pigs a.* A combination of streptomycin (IM) and streptomycin or nitrofurazone orally can also be used. None of these drugs, including terramycin, is completely effective
		b. Atrophic rhinitis (wasting away of the mucous membranes of the snout)		*Pigs b.* Sulfamethazine in the feed (50 mg/lb of feed cures the carrier animal in 3–5 weeks) or sodium sulfathiazole (0.5–0.66 gm/gal of drinking water) are also used
		c. Leptospirosis	*Pigs c.* 250 mg per each lb of feed for 14 days	*Pigs c.* Will reduce abortions caused by leptospirosis
		5. *Poultry:* a. Infectious synovitis (infectious arthritis)		*Poultry a.* Treatment with chlortetracycline is most effective. Terramycin is also used (in the feed)
		b. Erysipelas	*Poultry b.* Feed 200–250 mg per lb of feed	*Poultry b.* Each bird must be injected with *E. Insidiosa* bacterin at the same time
		c. Blue Comb disease	*Poultry c.* *Chickens.* 200–1,000 mg (equal to 1 gm) per gal of drinking water for a week or 50 mg per bird daily (in capsule form) given orally during a week. Follow either treatment with 100 mg mixed into each lb of feed during 2 weeks	

Drug	Uses	Dosage	Remarks
	d. Chronic respiratory disease	*Turkeys.* 1 mg per gal of drinking water. Do not give more than 5 days!	*Poultry d.* Tylosin is the most effective drug. Variation in treatment reaction is due to secondary bacterial invaders. If disease is serious, first inject, then mix drug into the feed or water 3–5 days
	6. *Newborn Animals* a. General disease preventative and growth stimulant	*Poultry d.* 50 mg per lb of feed *Newborn Animals a.* 2.5–12.5 mg per lb of feed *General Dosage:* Orally (*all farm animals except mature cattle, sheep, and goats*). 1.25–2.5 mg/lb body wt every 6 hours (*IV*), (*IM*) *and* (*SC*) *Injections* (*all farm animals*). 2–5 mg/lb body wt every 24 hours	*Toxic Reactions.* High oral doses will cause digestive problems in cattle, sheep, and goats. Injected cattle may go into shock and infrequently die
Neomycin	1. *All Species:* a. Bacterial infections of the intestines b. Wounds and infections of the skin, ears, and eyes.		*All Species a.* Given orally *All Species b.* Applied locally to the infected spot or wound
Polymixin	1. *All Species:* a. Infections of the skin, ears and eyes.		*All Species a.* May be used alone locally or mixed with Bacitracin or Neomycin

Class of Drug	Chemical Name (Common Name)	Disease	Dosage	Other Information
	Erythromycin (ilotycin)	1. *Pigs:* a. Infectious diarrhea	*Pigs a.* 25 mg given to piglets by (IM) injection within first 24 hrs after birth reduces cases of and deaths from the disease. To treat use 10 mg/lb body wt daily	
	Novobiocin (Albamycin, Cathomycin)			*Novobiocin.* Can be used when a microorganism is resistant to penicillin
	Tylosin	1. *Pigs:* a. Swine dysentery (bloody scours)	*Pigs a.* 1 gm per gal of drinking water 48 hrs, followed by 20–50 mg per lb of feed for 2–6 weeks afterward. If the disease reoccurs start the whole treatment over. The drinking water treatment can be replaced by an (IM) injection of 200 mg	*Poultry a.* Tylosin is the best drug but chlortetracycline, erythromycin, carbomycin, oxytetracycline, spiramycin, and streptomycin can be used instead
		2. *Poultry:* a. Chronic respiratory disease in chickens		
		b. Infectious sinusitis in turkeys	*Poultry b.* The bird is treated by having 1–6 mg injected into its sinuses	*Poultry b.* Tylosin is the best but the same drugs may be substituted as in chronic respiratory disease in chickens

Nitrofurans	Nitrofurazone (Furacin)	1. *All Farm Animals:* a. Bacterial surface infections or injuries to the skin, eyes, udder, and genitals	*All Farm Animals a.* Applied as a 0.2% ointment to the surface of the injury. Genital infections are treated with a 0.2% solution infused into the uterus	*All Farm Animals a.* Applied locally to the site. A suspension can also be used that contains a 2% mixture of nitrofurazone and procaine penicillin G
		2. *Pigs:* a. Infectious necrotic enteritis (pig typhoid)	*Pigs a.* Add 9 gm (of the 4.59% water-soluble powder) to each gal of drinking water	
		3. *Pigs and Cattle:* a. Intestinal salmonellosis infections (paratyphoid)	*Pigs and Cattle a.* 5 mg/lb body wt orally once daily for up to 6 days. Give the drug in water	

		4. *Poultry:*
		  a. Cecal coccidiosis of chickens
		  b. Intestinal coccidiosis of chickens
			Poultry a. Add 6.6 gm (of the 4.59% water-soluble powder) to each gal of drinking water
			Poultry b. Same treatment as cecal form
				Poultry a. Sulfamethazine and sulfaquinoxaline are more commonly used for treatment
				Poultry b. Same drugs are used as in cecal form
				
				Warning: Solutions of the 4.59% water-soluble nitrofurazone powder left in constant contact with metal for over 7 days will lose their effectiveness.

Class of Drug	Chemical Name (Common Name)	Disease	Dosage	Other Information
	Furazolidone (Furoxone)	1. *Pigs:* a. Bacterial enteritis (white scours)		*Pigs a.* Should be given in the drinking water. No drug is completely effective against this disease
		b. Infectious hemorrhagic enteritis		*Pigs b.* Should be given in the drinking water. No drug is completely effective against this disease
		2. *Rabbits:* a. Enteritis		*Rabbits a.* Same as in *Pigs a.* and b.
		b. Pneumonia (caused by pasteurella)		*Rabbits b.* Terramycin, chlortetracycline, penicillin, or a combination of penicillin and streptomycin can also be used
		3. *Poultry:* a. Coccidiosis b. Fowl typhoid	*Poultry b.* Treat with 100 mg per lb of feed	*Poultry a.* Sulfamethazine or sulfaquinoxaline are more commonly used for treatment
		c. Pullorum disease	*Poultry c.* Same dosage as with Fowl typhoid	
		d. Histomaniasis	*Poultry d.* To prevent the disease continuously mix 50 mg to each lb of feed For treatment mix 100 mg to each lb of feed for 2–3 weeks	
		e. Hexamitiasis	*Poultry e.* Same prevention and treatment as with histomaniasis	*Poultry e.* Only affects turkeys
		f. Infectious synovitis (infect. arthritis)		*Poultry f.* Best treatment is with chlortetracyline. Terramycin can also be used
		g. Parathyphoid	*Poultry g.* Treat with 100 mg per lb of feed	

Nihydrazone	1. *Poultry:* a. Pullorum disease b. Fowl thyphoid c. Paratyphoid d. Coccidiosis e. Histomaniasis f. Chronic respiratory disease	*Poultry:* Treat with 50 mg per lb of feed	*Poultry c.* Furazolidone is most commonly used. No drug completely eliminates infection *Poultry d.* Sulfamethazine and sulfaquinoxaline are most commonly used *Poultry f.* Tylosin is the most effective drug treatment
Furaltadone (Valsyn)	1. *Cattle:* a. Mastitis		*Cattle a.* May be used on dry or lactating cows
Nifuraldezone (Furamazone)	1. *Cattle:* a. Enteric bacterial infections of calves		
Nitrofurfuryl Methyl Ether (Furaspor)	1. *All Farm Animals:* a. Ringworm		*All Farm Animals a.* Applied (as a liquid once a day to the affected spot)

12

EXTERNAL PARASITES

Insects, fleas, lice, and ticks live on and get their nourishment from farm animals. These external parasites cause damage in several different ways:

1. They annoy and upset animals reducing the amount of feed that they consume.
2. Some types suck blood which weakens animals and creates the proper conditions for disease.
3. Other types lay their eggs on animals and, after hatching, the larvae feed on the animals flesh and body tissues.
4. Many flies and some ticks are carriers of diseases. When they bite an animal or suck its blood they pass along infectious microorganisms.

External parasites create tremendous losses for farmers by occasionally killing animals; by weakening their body defenses and overall condition; by slowing their growth; by causing them to consume more feed than normal to maintain themselves; by reducing the work they can do; and by lowering the amount and quality of the milk, flesh, wool, eggs, and hides they produce.

Ticks

Ticks injure livestock by sucking their blood, injecting a toxin, a poisonous substance, into the animal when it inserts its "head" through the skin prior to removing blood; by causing a wound through which secondary infections can enter; and by spreading disease between animals.

During their lives ticks pass through 4 different stages: the egg; the larva (the immature tick with 6 legs that hatches from the egg); the nymph (the 8-legged, still immature tick that develops from a larva and in time becomes an adult if conditions are right); and the adult.

After having developed, an adult female tick will suck blood from the animal it's attached to for 5–14 days in warm weather and a month or longer in cold weather. After mating with a male, usually while still on the animal, and being full of blood, the female is ready to lay eggs.

She leaves the animal and generally lays one batch of eggs over a period of 1–2 weeks, if the weather is warm. However, some females, like the fowl tick (see Figure 40), lay one batch of eggs, then return to the same or a different animal to suck more blood. Again, after filling with blood they drop off to lay another batch. This may happen several times. After laying eggs female ticks of all species die.

The incubation period of the egg (the time during which the larva, the immature tick, forms in the egg) is between 10 days to 3 months depending on the variety of tick. A six-legged larva hatches from the egg. For the life cycle of a tick to continue, the larva must attach itself to an animal and suck blood until it can't hold anymore. This takes between 2 days and 3 weeks, again according to the type.

At this point the first real differentiation between ticks is made. Some types of ticks remain on the same animal during all the different stages of their growth; they are called *one-host ticks*. Other kinds, called *three-host ticks,* drop off after filling with blood as a larva and later as a nymph. This type must attach itself to an animal three times in its life, once after hatching as a larva, the second time after turning into a nymph, and the third time after having become an adult.

After the larva has engorged with blood it stays where it is on the animal if it's a one-host tick. If it's a three-host tick it drops off. Now comes

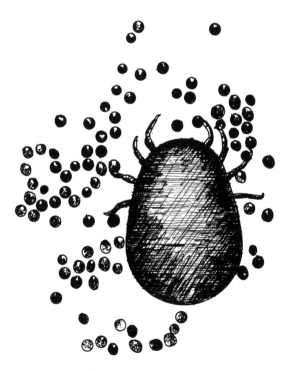

Figure 40.   Female fowl tick and its eggs.

an inactive time of 10 days to 3 weeks during which the six-legged larva develops into an eight-legged nymph.

If the nymph is a one-host tick it attaches in a different place on the same animal; if it's a three-host tick it must find a new animal to attach itself to within a number of months or it dies. Nymphs take as long as larvae do to fill up with blood but may need an inactive period of up to 3 months to transform themselves into adults.

The nymph of the one-host tick stays on the same animal; the nymph of the three-host tick drops off during this inactive period. Small nymphs become males and the larger ones turn into females.

After becoming an adult the female reattaches herself to the same animal (one-host tick) or a new animal (three-host tick), and begins to fill with blood. The male searches for a female with which to mate.

Tick Control and Treatment

Individual animals should be sprayed with a 0.5% solution of toxaphene (check manfacturer's instructions as to how to mix this with water) once every 2 weeks if they have 3-host ticks and once a month if they have 1-host ticks. You can use a 2–3 gallon hand-held or backpack sprayer for a couple of animals and a larger, commercial unit for a herd. Use cattle as a guide to estimate how much to spray. Short-haired cattle usually get 1 gallon, long-haired types get 2 gallons. Make sure you completely wet the animal to the skin no matter how much spray it takes!

For ear ticks spray the head, ears, and neck at low pressure. Treatment is once a month and from 1–2 pints per cow. There are several insec-

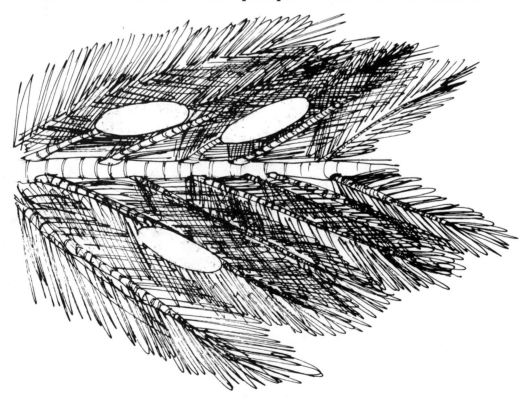

Figure 41.   Lice eggs attached to chicken feathers.

ticides that can be used for ear ticks, such as toxaphene, lindane, ronnel, coumaphos, or malathion. Check with your veterinary supply house as to what they have in stock and which is best for your type of animal.

An easy-to-perpare home remedy for ear ticks is a mixture of 2 parts of pine tar and 1 part of cottonseed oil applied directly into the ear with an oiling can. Treatment should be repeated every 2 weeks until animals are rid of ticks. Never let any of this mixture run down the animal's face as it will take the hair off.

In addition to treating tick infested animals, their housing must be completely sprayed with an insecticide at least twice a year. Use a 0.5% solution of toxaphene or lindane. Be sure you spray into all cracks and hiding places.

Never pull a tick off an animal by hand! Ticks suck blood by inserting their "head" through the skin and into the underlying flesh. If a tick is firmly attached and you pull it off, the head stays behind. Quite often these spots become infected or form abcesses. What you can do if an animal only has a few ticks and you don't want to go to the trouble of spraying it is to light a match and blow it out. Immediately put the hot stub of the match on the tick's blood-filled rear part. It will back its head out of the skin and the flesh below trying to get away from the heat. Now, just pick it off the animal's skin and squash or burn it.

Lice

Lice are flat parasitic insects that live on animals. There are two types: blood-sucking and biting (those that live from the pieces of skin, scales, or hair they bite off and eat).

These little parasites, between an eighth and a quarter of an inch when fully grown, cause itching and irritation. The animal rubs itself on posts, trees, or buildings in an effort to stop the itching. This in turn opens wounds, perfect spots for secondary invasion by infections or other pests and parasites, and also damages fleeces in sheep and goats. Blood-sucking lice often cause anemia and lower milk production and growth rates.

Female lice lay oval-shaped, yellowish-white eggs. They attach them to the animal's hairs, bristles, or feathers (see Figure 41), in and around the ear, on the shoulders, the neck, and the inside of the legs close to the underbelly. In sheep a particular kind of louse, called the foot louse, attaches its eggs to the coarse hairs above the hooves around the dew claws. In a heavy infestation they may extend all the way up the legs to the abdomen.

Eggs closest to the body hatch first, because of body heat, and are called nymphs, the immature stage of the louse. Eggs generally hatch in 1–3 weeks depending on the species and weather conditions. The nymph stage lasts 11–21 days after which the lice are mature and the males and females mate. Females begin to lay eggs shortly afterwards.

Sucking lice are blue or dark gray in color with long pointed heads. Biting lice are yellow or reddish-brown and have short broad heads. See Figures 42 and 43 to note the difference between biting and bloodsucking lice in cattle. Figures 44 (blood-sucking louse of the horse, mule, and donkey), 45 (the female biting sheep louse), 46 (the blood-sucking pig louse), and 47 (the male head louse in chickens) will be of help in identifying these pests.

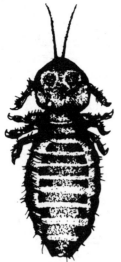

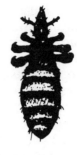

Figure 43.   **The blood sucking louse of the cow.**

Figure 42.   **The biting louse of the cow.**

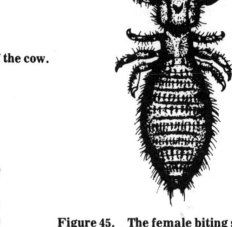

Figure 45.   **The female biting sheep louse.**

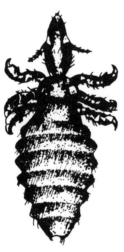

Figure 44.   **The blood sucking louse of the horse, mule, and donkey.**

Lice Control and Treatment

Horses, Mules, Donkeys, and Cattle

When one animal is discovered to have lice you must assume all of its herdmates are affected as well. Treat all animals.

If you have small numbers of animals the easiest lice treatment is to spray on an effective insecticide using a 2-3 gallon hand-held pressure sprayer, at very low pressure, or to apply an insecticidal powder by hand. Whichever method you use make sure the insecticide is evenly distributed over the animal's entire body. Be sure to cover the tail, underarms, around the anus, vagina, and hooves, and the head area, especially the inner ears.

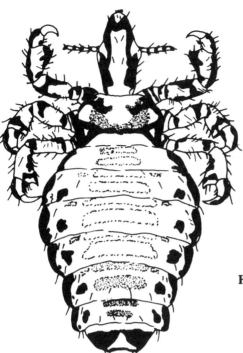

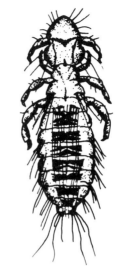

Figure 47.   The male head louse of the chicken.

Figure 46.   The blood sucking pig louse.

Before spraying make sure animals are not overheated and that the weather is warm, otherwise they're liable to be chilled. Dusting is used during cold weather.

Some of the common chemical products for both spraying and dusting are toxaphene, lindane, and chlordane. Natural insecticides, produced from plant products, are rotenone (made from derris root) and pyrethrin (made from the flower pyrethrum).

Pigs

Pigs can be treated by covering their entire bodies with a thin coat of used crankcase oil. Or if you don't have a supply of oil, make a kerosene emulsion (a mixture in which an oil is distributed in another liquid). To do this cut one-half pound of soap in little pieces and place into 1 gallon of water. Heat the water until the soap dissolves. Then pour in 2 gallons of kerosene and stir and mix it well until there is no free-standing kerosene left on top of the water. Dilute this mixture by adding 11 gallons of water. Now you are ready to swab down those hogs.

Freshly oiled pigs should be kept out of bright sunlight, shouldn't be forced to move too quickly, and must be protected from chilling for a day or two. They need plenty of shade.

Pig oilings can be supplemented by driving a post into the ground and wrapping it with old rags or burlap sacks. Soak the rags and sacks with crankcase oil periodically, and as your pigs scratch they'll self-oil themselves (see Figure 48). Piglets can be treated by filling a small barrel with used oil and dipping their entire bodies. Grasp them just above the hooves of the front legs and lower them into the barrel hindquarters first (see Figure 49).

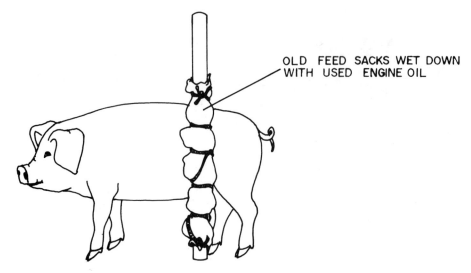

Figure 48.   An oiling post to control lice in pigs.

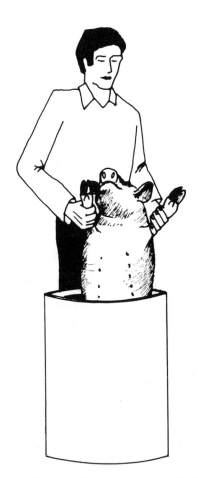

Figure 49.   Oil piglets by dipping them in a barrel filled with used engine oil.

Sheep and Goats

Dipping vats are generally used to treat lice infestations of sheep and goats. The vat is a round or rectangular concrete pit constructed in the ground. The pit drops off sharply at one end to a depth of 54 inches and rises gradually at the other end so the animal can walk out under its own power (see Figures 50 and 51). The vat should be long enough so the animal has to swim from one end to the other. If you have lots of animals make it long enough so that a good number can be dipped at the same time.

Both goats and sheep should be kept in the dipping vat about 1 minute, just long enough to thoroughly wet their wool and skin. The animal is carefully thrown into the vat or worked through a chute, which has been filled to a depth of 40–48 inches so that its whole body submerges. When it comes to the surface give it time to catch its breath, then push the animal's head under the dip solution with a pole. Do this once more before you let it climb out.

In order to estimate the amount of insecticide solution to fill the dipping vat with, you should know that freshly sheared goats and sheep carry out 2 quarts of liquid. Before shearing and when their fleece is long they carry out 1 gallon apiece.

Dipping should never be done when the animal is overheated, the day too hot or when it will turn cold before the goat or sheep can dry off. If animals must be herded long distances to be brought to the dipping vat give them a day to rest and calm down before being treated.

Lindane, dioxathion, toxaphene, coumaphos, ronnel, rotenone, and crufomate are all chemicals that can be used for the dip solution. Always check the manufacturer's instructions for mixing proportions. For milk goats use only crotoxyphos, coumaphos, or rotenone as other chemicals leave a residue in the milk.

In cold or winter weather when it's not possible to dip, use a dry powder. Make sure it's rubbed onto the animal's entire body including the insides of the ears and the underarms. Only the three chemicals mentioned

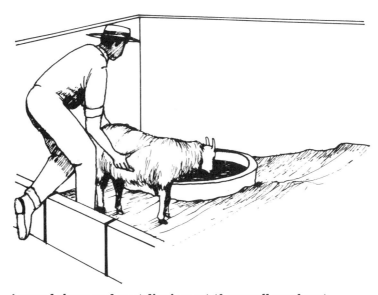

Figure 50.   A round sheep and goat dipping vat (for small numbers).

above can be used on milking goats. Other goats and sheep can receive coumaphos, diazinon, crotoxyphos, and methexychlor in powder form.

Poultry

With small numbers of birds the best treatment is the "pinch method." The chicken is held in one hand; grasp both wings at their base, close to the body, and hold them together behind the bird's back. With the other hand apply pinches of sodium fluoride, a poisonous insecticide, to different parts of the body.

A pinch is the amount of powder you can hold between your thumb and first finger. Apply 11 pinches: one each placed on the head, breast, neck, tail, vent, each thigh, and each wing; the back gets 2 pinches.

Sodium fluoride is poisonous. Wear a wet handkerchief or commercial mask over your nose and mouth so as not to breathe in the dust. After treating your birds wash your hands and arms thoroughly in soap and water and store the remaining sodium fluoride in a secure place. Safeguard it from curious children. Clearly label the container so you don't mistake it for something else and use it accidentally.

It's a good idea to delouse hens before their chicks hatch because the insecticide will injure the chicks while they hover under their mothers to keep warm. If the sodium fluoride doesn't kill the chicks, lice will, so make sure hens are deloused. Turkeys, because they're bigger, are treated with 15 pinches; ducks get 11 pinches, the same amount as chickens.

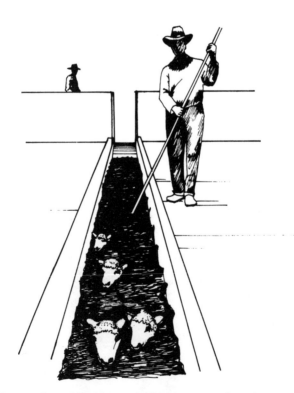

Figure 51.   A sheep and goat dipping vat (for large numbers).

Dipping Schedule

Lice eggs hatch at different times depending on how far from the animal's body they are (which determines how much body heat they receive), and according to weather conditions. In cold weather eggs hatch more slowly than when it's warm and sunny. As a result several dippings are necessary to rid an animal of most of its lice. Even then you're never sure you've killed them all, so examine your animals frequently.

First Dipping—should be done in moderately warm weather
Second Dipping—12-14 days later
Third Dipping—17-21 days after the first dipping

If you can't get in three dippings because of adverse weather try 2 dippings 17-21 days apart. If after the first dip the weather turns cold, you may have to dust instead for the following external parasites. Use the same schedules for treatment whether dipping, spraying, or dusting.

Fleas

The adult female flea lays her oval white eggs on an animal's skin, usually that of a dog, cat, or pig. The eggs drop to the ground and after several days hatch out as larvae. These look like tiny worms. The larvae live on bits of organic matter to be found in the ground. One of their favorite spots is where animals sleep.

After about 2 weeks the larvae have become full grown and spin cocoons around themselves. While inside the cocoons—about the size of a grain of wheat—the larvae turn into pupae. The pupa is a stage the immature flea passes through before becoming a mature adult (see Figure 52). Within a week after transforming itself into a pupa, the flea develops into an adult.

Fleas live on animal's blood and are carriers of other parasites and diseases. They irritate and cause uneasiness in animals which results in time being lost from eating, reduced weight gains, and lowered milk production. Animals may rub themselves against posts or other objects in an attempt to relieve the itching caused by flea bites.

Flea Control and Treatment

Treat animal's backs, necks, and heads with derris powder (since it contains rotenone), pyrethrum powders, or rotenone itself. These few spots are sufficient as fleas move extensively over an animal's body. Pigs

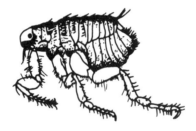

Figure 52.   The adult flea.

can be treated by wetting their backs with crankcase oil. Chickens are generally not treated directly but their coops are disinfected by spraying them with a strong insecticide. Check with a veterinary supply store for a recommended product.

Mites

Mites are extremely tiny parasites, sometimes visible to the eye when held against a dark background. They are more easily seen when looked at under a magnifying glass. These eight-legged creatures cause scabies, a contagious disease of the surface of the skin, and mange, also called scab, a skin disease of the tissue under the outer surface. The symptoms in all species of farm animals are the same: inflammation, intense itching, scratching, rubbing, and biting of affected areas of the skin.

There are two general types of scabies-causing mites: psoroptic and chorioptic; and three kinds of mange-causing mites: sarcoptic, demodectic, and psorergatic. The following is a description of each type.

Psoroptic Scabies

Psoroptic scabies is caused by a miniscule mite that lives its entire life on the animal. The female lays 15–25 eggs on the skin which hatch in 4 days. These little immature mites—the larvae—have 3 pairs of legs. They become nymphs, which in turn develop into adults with 4 pairs of legs. Males and females mate, then 2 days later the new generation of females begins laying eggs. The whole process takes 16 days from egg laying to egg laying.

Psoroptic mites are common to horses, mules, cattle, sheep, and goats. They attack hairy parts of the body in general. By species they will be found in colonies in the following places: horse and mule—under the mane, the beginning of the tail, and the crown and back of the head; cattle—the beginning of the tail, on the back, and the withers (the point of the back found by continuing an imaginary line straight up from the shoulders); sheep and goats—on the back and sides.

The adult mites have pointed mouth parts (see Figure 53) which they use to puncture the skin and suck blood serum. The serum oozes out of the puncture openings and mixes with dried skin, dust, and other dirt. This mixture dries and forms a crusty scab. The skin becomes hard, leathery, and wrinkled; occasionally it will crack and bleed when folded, rubbed, scratched, or bitten. Hair and wool fall out leaving grayish bare spots. The mites spread the scabies by moving away from this zone of injured skin toward more healthy areas. Here they repeat the whole process.

Chorioptic Scabies

Chorioptic scabies, also called foot scabies, is caused by a mite very similar to the psoroptic mite. They're distinguished by the location on the body where they are found. Chorioptic mites are found in the following

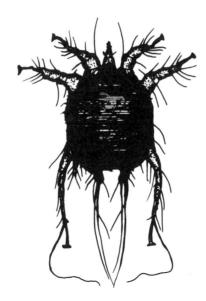

Figure 53.   The adult male psoroptic mite.

places: horses and mules—the lower legs below the knees and hocks; cattle—the insides of the hind legs and the upper, rear part of the udder and scrotum; sheep and goats—around the feet, the inner sides of the legs, the udder, and the abdomen.

Chorioptic mites pierce the skin causing blood serum and tissue fluids to ooze out of the wound. These fluids form blisters that merge and burst. The dried material that's left forms crusty scabs that build up over time. The mites live in groups under the scabs where the skin is very irritated and bleeds easily.

Sarcoptic Mange

In sarcoptic mange the adult female mite burrows through the upper layer of the skin into underlying tissue. She begins to lay eggs almost as soon as she enters the burrow and will continue to deposit them for up to 2 months. In total she lays 25–30 eggs that hatch within 5 days.

The larvae leave the burrow to live and develop on the skin. Here they go through the nymph stage and become adult males and females. The mites mate on the skin surface and the now fertilized female begins her own burrow and starts to lay eggs. From egg laying to egg laying takes 2 weeks (see Figure 54).

In general, sarcoptic mites attack tender, thin-skinned areas of the body that have little hair cover. They are found in the following places: horses and mules—at first on the head, neck, and shoulders, but afterward all over the body; cattle—high up on the rear of the udder and scrotum, the backs and inner parts of the thighs, the beginning of the tail and the lower neck; sheep and goats—the head and face; pigs—the head, especially around the eyes and snout, inside the ears, and on the hind legs.

As the mites burrow through and eat the animal's tissue this injury causes swelling, irritation, and terrible itching. With rubbing, itching, and biting the hair falls out. The skin becomes thick, hardened, and full of

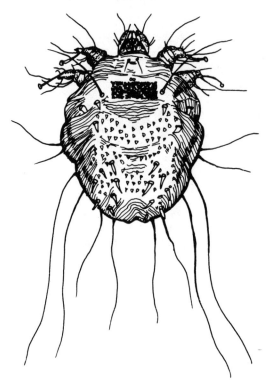

Figure 54.   The female sarcoptic mange mite.

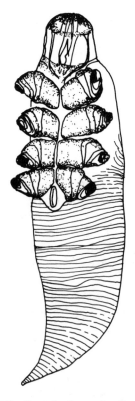

Figure 55.   The female demodectic mange mite.

scabs. Dandruff is a common sign. The skin cracks, and blood and pus are seen.

Milk cows with sarcoptic mange may develop mastitis or inflamed udders as a result of rubbing and scratching their udders.

Demodectic Mange

Demodectic mange is caused by a slow-moving, microscopic mite with a body the shape of a cigar. This mite causes rounded lumps (nodules) under the skin that vary in size from the head of a pin to a walnut. These lumps fill with a cheesy white pus that sometimes oozes out onto the skin surface when they break and are squeezed or cut open.

The demodectic mite is found in the following places: cattle—the neck, brisket (the chestbone), and shoulders; sheep—in the glands of the eyelids; goats—the bottom of the hips, the flanks (the area just in front of the hind legs and above the udder), and around the ears and jaws; pigs—at first on the snout and around the eyelids, but later it spreads to the underpart of the neck, the breast area, the abdomen, and insides of the legs. The mite likes to attack the animal where its skin is tender and thin (see Figure 55).

Psorergatic Mange

Psorergatic mites are round in shape with double hooks on their legs adapted to burrowing. They burrow under the skin, causing irritation and itching that the animal tries to alleviate by rubbing, scratching, and biting. The skin becomes rough, thick, and scaly. The scabs that form are dry, loose on the surface, and crumbly.

Sheep are the only common farm animal affected by the psorergatic mite.

Chicken Mites

Two general types of mites affect chickens and, to a lesser extent, turkeys. The first kind spends most of its time in the chickenhouse hidden in cracks and crevices, coming out at night to suck blood from the birds. The second type, of which there are several varieties, lives its entire life on the bird. These mites are found on the vent (the bird's anus), the parts of the legs without feathers, and on the back and sides, burrowed into the skin at the base of the feathers.

The signs of infestation are irritation and redness of the vent with dirty feathers around it, swollen feet and legs that may lose their scales, and plenty of scabs on the skin of the back and sides, as well as feathers that fall out or break off.

Chicken mites cause slow growth, anemia, reduced egg production, death in some chicks and laying birds, and they transmit serious diseases, such as fowl cholera and Newcastle disease.

Rabbit Mites

The most common rabbit mites (psoroptic and chorioptic) attack the inside of the ears. You'll know your animals are infested when you notice them shaking their heads, flapping their ears, and scratching at them with their hind feet.

Affected rabbits lose weight and are often attacked by secondary infections. The mites cause the oozing of blood serum and body fluids; crusty scabs form on the lining of the inner part of the ear.

Rabbits are also attacked by two different mites that cause mange. Animals scratch themselves constantly and lose hair from the nose, chin, head, and around the eyes and ears. Rabbit mange is very contagious and it's important to separate infested animals from their herdmates as soon as the symptoms are noticed.

Mite Control and Treatment

The prevention of mite infestation is based on good management. Animal housing and quarters must be kept clean by a regular disinfection schedule, the animals should be groomed and kept clean (in the horse and mule this means disinfection of blankets and saddles, as well) and they must be fed a well-balanced diet. Healthy animals maintained in clean housing and surroundings are less frequently attacked by mites than those that are sick or in a weakened condition and kept in dirty, unsanitary environments.

Psoroptic and Chorioptic Scabies and Psorergatic Mange

Dip or spray the animal twice, 10–12 days apart. Make sure the entire body is wet and, when dipped, that the animal's head submerges twice. Animals should be kept in the dip vat for at least one minute. Before dipping, hard scabs must be softened or soaked with the dip solution so that it penetrates and reaches the mites underneath.

Use solutions of rotenone, lindane, or benzene hexachloride (BHC) to dip or spray with, according to the manufacturer's instructions. Freshly dipped animals must be kept out of the sun and wind for a few hours so the insecticide has a chance to soak in. In cold or wet weather apply insecticide powders or dusts instead of dipping or spraying.

Sarcoptic Mange

Since sarcoptic mites burrow under the skin and are hard to reach with insecticides, animals should be dipped 3-4 times, 6–10 days apart. Use spray and dip solutions of lindane, nicotine sulfate, or BHC according to the manufacturer's instructions. The procedure is the same as with psoroptic, chorioptic, and psorergatic mites. In cold or wet weather animals should be dusted with lindane, BHC powders, or dusts. Dust litter and bedding as well.

Demodectic Mange

A wash of lindane or BHC (the strength should be determined according to the manufacturer's instructions) is used to kill demodectic mites in open nodules. If the nodules are large and not yet open, cut them open with a sterilized knife or razor blade. Squeeze out the contents (and burn them) and apply tincture of iodine. A lindane or BHC wash can be used instead.

If the nodules are infected or have formed abscesses, wash them out with soap and water, then swab them with a piece of clean, sterile cotton soaked in iodine.

Chicken Mites

Chickens are rid of mites according to the specific type. For mites that live in the chickenhouse and suck the bird's blood at night, the entire chickenhouse is disinfected twice, 10-12 days apart, with lindane or malathion, according to the manufacturer's instructions. Litter is burned and the manure is removed from the floor and scraped from roosts. Lindane or malathion can also be painted on the roosts.

For mites that attack the vent, the bird can be dusted or dipped with sulfur. The dip is prepared by mixing 2 ounces of finely ground sulfur (the specific kind is called 325 mesh, which refers to the fineness of its particles) and 1 ounce of any kind of detergent soap powder in 1 gallon of warm water. The bird must be wet to the skin (of course, including its feathers) and have its head submerged in the solution. Dip on a warm day as many times as necessary.

Mites that infest the legs are eliminated by dipping the bird's feet and legs up to the feather line in used crankcase oil. Dip twice, 1 month apart.

For mites that burrow into the skin at the base of the feathers, birds must be dipped in a wettable sulfur solution mixed in water. (A wettable solution is one that has had a chemical added that makes it mix more easily with water.) Prepare the dip by mixing 2 ounces of wettable sulfur in 1 gallon of warm water. Dip the bird several times, 6-10 days apart.

Rabbit Mites

Before treating ear mites the crumbly scabs that line the inner ear must be removed. Hold the animal firmly, then dip a piece of clean, sterile cotton in hydrogen peroxide (a cleaning agent) diluted in water. Remove the scabs by washing out the ears with the cotton-filled mixture. After this cleaning, swab out the ears with a mixture of 1 part Canex, which contains a combination of chloroform, rotenone, and other extracts from derris root, and 3 parts mineral or vegetable oil. Pour the mixture into the ear as far as it goes, so that it reaches the inner ear, and wet the area around the ear, the head, and the neck. Repeat the treatment in 6-10 days. The hutch must be well disinfected.

When the rabbit is affected by mites on any other part of the body it's dipped into a lime-sulfur solution (usually 1 quart of the lime-sulfur solution is diluted with 4 gallons of water, but check the manufacturer's instructions) or Canex is rubbed into the mite-infested skin. If you use the lime-sulfur dip repeat the treatment in 6-10 days.

A Warning about Lindane and BHC Use

Milk products (milk, cheese, butter, and yogurt) from cattle and goats that are sprayed with, dipped in, or dusted with lindane or BHC cannot be used for human consumption for to 3–4 days after treatment. A small amount of these insecticides is absorbed through the skin and ends up in the animal's tissues from which it passes into the milk. The milk can be fed to calves, kids, and pigs during this period.

Any animal that will be slaughtered for meat must not have been dipped, sprayed, or dusted during the preceding 30 days. After treatment small amounts of lindane and BHC remain in the animal's tissues for that time period. Eating meat that contains minute quantities of these insecticides can cause sickness.

Both lindane and BHC must be removed from dipping vats and disposed of in a place that animals cannot reach and that is not used for grazing. Small pools or puddles should not be allowed to collect as animals may drink from them and this would be very dangerous. Both these insecticides poison fish and should never be dumped into or near streams, rivers, or lakes.

13

MORE EXTERNAL PARASITES

Flies

Flies cause losses in many ways to animal-raisers. They bite and suck animals' blood, weakening their resistance to disease. They annoy and irritate animals, which causes them to lose time from eating and lowers their food intake, growth, and milk production.

Flies are carriers of many diseases and some internal parasites which they transmit from animal to animal. They lay eggs on the animal which may then swallow them. The eggs hatch, and as the larvae pass through the animal's system they injure various organs and eat tissue. Some larvae may eat flesh at the surface, usually in open wounds. Other kinds, after hatching, are capable of burrowing through the animal's skin, and again, eating tissue and weakening its condition.

Mosquitoes

Mosquitoes (see Figures 56a and b) suck blood, often causing anemia, and transmit a number of diseases, such as equine encephalo-myelitis (a virus that attacks the brain and spinal cord of horses and mules). Because of the annoyance that mosquitoes cause, animals don't gain as much weight or produce as much milk as they would normally.

The larvae grow in stagnant pools, wet spots in fields, where water stands for some time or moves very slowly, and in swamps and marshes (see Figure 57). Unless mosquito larvae control is practiced on a community-wide basis it is impractical to attempt to do so as an individual. Standing water must be eliminated and animals checked frequently to see if they are being attacked. If so, spray or dust them with a natural insecticide, such as pyrethrum.

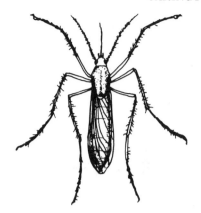

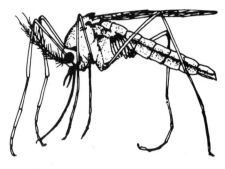

Figure 56b.   Mosquito (side view).

Figure 56a.   Mosquito (top view).

Gnats

Gnats come in two varieties, the blackfly, a small, dark-colored fly with a rounded back (see Figure 58) and the sandfly, a much tinier, gray-black fly with spots on its wings.

The blackfly sucks blood and passes along diseases and parasites. One of the parasites, the filaria worm, can cause blindness in animals and humans. Sandflies also transmit disease and their bites are painful. Control both of these pests by dusting or spraying animals daily with pyrethrum during outbreaks.

Horseflies and Deer Flies

Horseflies and deer flies range in size from ½-1½ inches. (see Figures 59–60). They make painful cuts in an animal's skin from which they suck its blood and through which they transmit dangerous diseases like anthrax and anaplasmosis.

Control of these two flies is extremely difficult. Luckily, they only appear for short periods of time during the year. Spray animals with a synergized pyrethrum emulsion at the rate of 1 quart per animal. Protection last 3 days.

Houseflies

Houseflies (see Figure 61) don't bite or suck blood, but they do carry all sorts of infectious organisms and matter. They feed on eye secretions and are an intermediate host and transmitter of ascarids, also called *round worms* (an internal parasite), in horses and mules.

Houseflies develop in manure, filth, garbage, and decay products. Housing should be disinfected regularly, manure spread or composted, and garbage cleaned up.

Bait made of powdered malathion or other products mixed with liquid sugar, honey, or molasses are used when housefly numbers

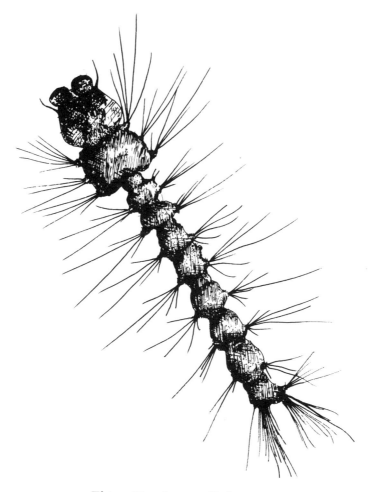

Figure 57. A mosquito larva.

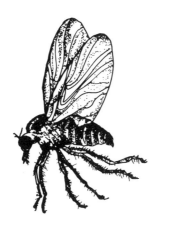

Figure 58. The black fly.

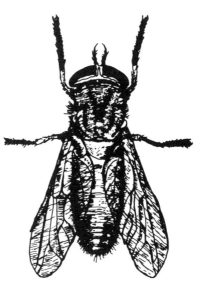

Figure 59. The horse fly.

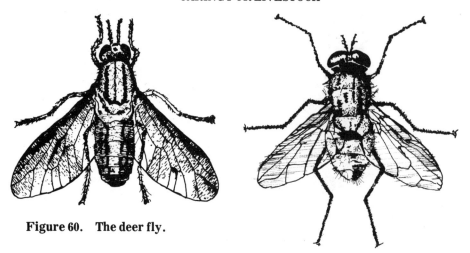

Figure 60.   The deer fly.

Figure 61.   The house fly.

become too great. Put the bait into pans and the flies will be attracted by the sweetness. Make sure they're put in inaccessible places where neither children nor small animals can reach them.

Hornflies

Hornflies (see Figure 62) attack cattle, sucking blood from around the horns (where they spend most of their time), the back, shoulders, and abdomen. They're half the size of houseflies and only leave the animal when laying their eggs in its manure.

Beef cattle should be sprayed with methoxyclor, malathion, toxaphene, or pyrethrum. The first three insecticides are effective for 3 weeks following a spraying; pyrethrum offers protection for 3-7 days. Because these chemicals pass into the milk in dairy cattle they're not

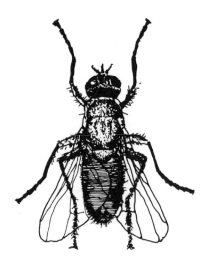

Figure 62.   The horn fly.

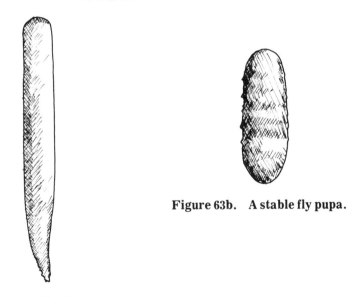

Figure 63b.   A stable fly pupa.

Figure 63a.   A stable fly larva.

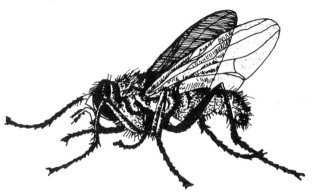

Figure 63c.   The adult stable fly.

recommended for treating them; instead use an oil spray of coumaphos, dichlorvos, or crotoxyphos.

Another treatment is to drive a post into the ground and wrap it with burlap bags that have been soaked with a mixture of insecticide and oil. The animals rub themselves against it and automatically apply the mixture.

Stable Flies

Stable flies look very much like houseflies (see Figures 63 a, b, and c) but have one of the most painful bites of any bloodsucking fly that attacks farm animals. The bites continue to bleed after the stable fly has left and are perfect sites for secondary attack by screwworm flies, houseflies, and other insects.

Stable flies cause losses by annoying animals and sucking blood; in severe attacks animals may die. They also transmit diseases such as anthrax. More normally, food intake is lowered, weight gains are reduced, and milk production decreases. The favorite places of attack are as follows: in horses, mules, cattles, sheep, and goats—the lower parts of the body, especially the outer sides of the front legs; in pigs and rabbits— the ears.

Since stable flies normally only suck blood from an animal once a day in wintertime and twice a day during the summer, it's hard to control them by spraying the animal. However, synergized pyrethrum or crotoxyphos sprays are recommended because they kill flies so quickly. Several products that give good results are synergized crotoxyphos, for example, ciodrin (use 1-2 quarts per cow, and don't apply more than once a week) or ciodrin-vapona oil base spray (not more than 2 ounces per animal, but it can be applied daily) and synergized pyrethrums, which can be applied daily but no more than 2 ounces per animal. Regardless of which spray you use it should be applied to the favorite stable fly-feeding sites on the animal, depending on what species you want to treat.

Barns and housing should be sprayed with ronnel, fenthion, dimethoate, rabon, or diazinon.

Screwworms

Screwworms are the larvae of a type of blowfly, which is also called the *screwworm fly* (see Figure 64). Screwworms develop in the tissues of living animals, whereas the larvae of other types of blow flies live on dead flesh.

The blue-green screwworm fly lays 200-400 eggs at one time (in total up to 3,000) alongside a wound. Within 12 hours the larvae hatch and immediately crawl to the wound and burrow into it. They live on body fluids and live tissue for about 6 days. At the end of this period they've turned a pink color and are now fully grown larvae.

The maggots leave the wounds, drop to the ground, and burrow under the surface where they develop into pupae. This inactive period lasts 8-60 days, depending on the temperature, after which time the new generation of screwworm flies emerges.

Screwworms don't like cold weather. In warm weather the whole life cycle will be completed within 21 days; in cold weather it can take up to

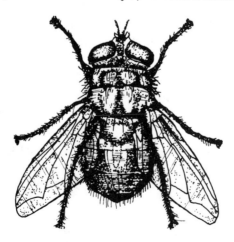

Figure 64.   The adult screw worm fly (also called the blow fly).

90. If temperatures drop below 50°F for 3 months in a row or if the temperature reaches freezing even once, screwworm flies and larvae, at whatever stage of their development, will die.

The larvae look like screws; the front part of the 12 millimeter-long body is pointed, the rear part wider and blunt. Screwworms feed together as a group. In the event that a heavily infested animal is not treated within 2 weeks, it is almost certain to die.

Wounds being attacked by screwworms ooze a lot of reddish-brown fluid that usually stains the surrounding hair or wool. Animals become restless, annoyed, are off feed, separate themselves from the herd, and try to hide in dense brush to get away from the attack of screwworm flies, blowflies, houseflies, and other insects that feed on the fluid discharge from their wounds.

Prevention

Since screwworm flies lay their eggs on the edge of wounds, the best prevention is to control wounds and injury during fly season. Where screwworms are a problem, don't castrate or dock tails by the incision method (using a knife) but instead use an emasculatome or elastration ring (see Chapter 17, Minor Operations, the section on "Castration," p. 209).

Control your breeding schedule so that animals are not born during fly season (usually warm weather). The navel and umblilical cord are favorite screwworm places of attack. If young are born during fly season treat these two areas with EQ-335, a screwworm insecticide. Be careful to follow the manufacturer's instructions about dosage, as lindane, the drug used as the basis of EQ-335, can be harmful to young animals.

Animals with wounds, no matter how small, must have them treated immediately with an antiseptic and then should have a screwworm remedy applied. See the next section, "Treatment," for the specific product. Since fly and tick wounds are also possible screwworm attack sites, eliminate these parasite pests from your animals on a regular basis.

Treatment

There are several products that have been developed in the last 30 years, mostly by the U.S. Department of Agriculture, with which you can effectively treat your animals after they've been infested with screwworms and to protect them against future attacks.

EQ-335, a solution that contains lindane as its killing agent, can be bought from a verterinary supply house or made at home. If you have many animals it may be cheaper to make it yourself, but make sure this is true by checking ingredient prices.

EQ-335 is made by accurately weighing all ingredients and mixing them together. Add 3 parts of lindane, 35 parts of pine oil, 42 parts of white mineral oil, 10 parts of any emulsifier (an agent that holds an oily liquid suspended in another fluid), and 10 parts of silica gel. EQ-335 contains 3 percent lindane; any other product used to treat screwworms that has between 3-5 percent lindane in it will work just as well.

Smear 62 is a screwworm remedy that uses benzene, a clear,

poisonous liquid, as the killing agent instead of lindane. Another product uses the insecticide ronnel to kill screwworms.

All three of these smears are interchangeable. If you can't get a supply of one, try another. Paint them on the wound with a small, 1-inch-wide paint brush. Be sure you reach all the folds of the wound and areas the maggots have burrowed into. Also paint the skin right around the wound.

You can also dust wounds with a powder that contains 5 percent coumaphos or spray them with coumaphos or ronnel. These should kill existing larvae and prevent further infestation for 2 weeks.

Blowflies

Blowflies are very similar to screwworm flies, with 2 differences: their color, which varies from green to black, always has a metallic sheen to it and they lay their eggs on dead animals, which supply the main food source for the developing larvae.

Control

Blowfly larvae are controlled by burning the carcasses of dead animals. Dig a pit alongside the animal, fill it with wood, roll the animal on top, and set the whole pile on fire. The entire body must be completely burned. But never burn a carcass when an animal has died of anthrax, the spores will be spread by the smoke. See Chapter 16, General Diseases of Domestic Animals, "Treatment of the Carcass," p.172.

If the dead body has lain unburned for more than 2 days , it's possible that some of the larvae have completed their cycle and have burrowed into the ground in order to become pupae. If this is the case, shovel the hot coals in a circle 3 yards wide from where the dead body lay. The heat should kill any burrowing larvae.

During blowfly outbreaks animals should be sprayed or dusted in the same way as for screwworm flies. Blowflies may be killed during heavy infestations by putting out poison bait. Put a piece of meat in a pan partially filled with a poisonous solution of one-half an ounce of nicotine sulfate mixed into 1 gallon of water. Skim the dead flies off the surface of the poison. Be sure no animals can reach the bait as it will kill them just as well as the flies.

Wool Maggots

A few types of blowflies lay their eggs in sheeps' wool. They are attracted by the dirty, manure-filled wool around the anus and the odor produced by fermenting wool close to the skin during hot weather after a rain.

At first the larvae eat wool, but then move onto the skin and into the flesh (like their cousin, the screwworm). Wool maggot attacks spread quickly, within a week the animal's entire body may be infested, and are hard to recognize because the maggots feed below the surface of the wool.

Control

It is a good idea to shear sheep during blowfly season and then dip them. If it isn't possible, at least shear the wool between the legs and around the tail and anus. One insecticidal dipping with coumaphos, dioxathion, ronnel, or diazinon will protect your sheep for 6–8 weeks.

Previously existing wounds should be treated with EQ-335 or 1–2 ounces in total, per animal of 0.5 percent coumaphos dust once a week until they heal. Don't dust with coumaphos for at least 15 days before slaughtering an animal.

Once a animal has been attacked by wool maggots shear off the wool around the area and then paint on EQ-335 or Smear 62.

Cattle Grubs: Life Cycle

Cattle grubs, also called *ox warbles*, are the larvae of the heel fly, a hairy, fast-flying, black-and-yellow-striped cattle pest the size of a honeybee (see Figure 65). The fly gets its name from the part of the cow's body it's most often seen around (while it chases and terrorizes it) and where it lays its small, creamy white eggs (see Figure 66).

The eggs hatch into barely visible larvae within 2–6 days, crawl down the hair they were laid on, and burrow through the animal's skin into its tissue. For the next several months they move through the cow's connective tissue by secreting enzymes which dissolve the soft tissue, providing them with food. After a 2–4-month stationary growth period, either in the esophagus or spinal canal, depending on the specie of larvae, they reach the tissue that lies just under the skin of the back. There they create a hole in the skin, again by secreting enzymes, through which they breathe.

The body responds by forming cysts around the larvae (see Figure 67), which are seen as heavy lumps under the skin. The larvae irritate the cyst walls and live on the serum that bathes them, as well as on the secondary bacterial invaders. During the next 40–60 days the larvae continue to grow; they molt twice and finally emerge from their casings and drop to the ground. There they develop into pupae, the stationary, nonfeeding stage in the insects' lives in between the immature larvae and the adult heel flies. The pupae quickly acquire dark-colored, hard protective cases and are found in the soil or in scattered trash.

The cattle grub pupae are now 25 times the size of the eggs that were laid on the cow by the heel fly. They measure 1-inch long × ⅛-inch in diameter and have become dark gray-brown in color. In 1–3 months the mature heel flies emerge from their pupae cases, mate, and spend the rest of the 1 week of life that remains to them chasing and laying their eggs on cattle.

Signs of Attack and Infestation

On warm, sunny days when cattle, for no apparent reason, run wildly, in great fear and with their tails held high in the air, it's quite possible they're being attacked by heel flies. If that's the case, the cattle will

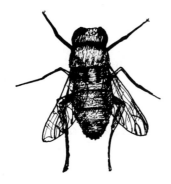

Figure 65.   The heel fly.

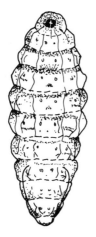

Figure 67.   The cattle grub larva.

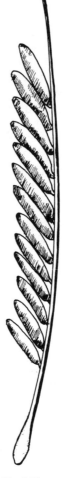

Figure 66.   Heel fly eggs laid on a hair.

head for the nearest shade, pond, river, or standing water where the flies won't pursue them.

The places where the larvae have burrowed through the animal's skin into its tissue will be recognized easily: they'll be inflamed, painful to the touch and usually seep a yellow serum. Larvae cysts just under the skin of the back are also unmistakable. They look like swollen lumps raised well above the normal level of the skin and may range from the shoulders to the beginning of the tail, along the back, and as far as one-third of the way down the animal's sides. The breathing holes are often abscessed and exude serum.

Treatment

Cattle are effectively treated for grubs by using systemic insecticides which kill the harmful larvae wherever they are in the animal's bodies. However, great caution must be exercised to treat the larvae at the proper stage of their development, and for your own safety, or disastrous results may occur (see the following section, ''Grub Treatment Warnings.''

Method of Treatment	Insecticide	Dosage	Other Indications
Pour-on	Coumaphos 4% solution	½ fluid oz per 100 lb body wt	
	Fenthion 3% solution	½ fluid oz per 100 lb body wt	
	Fenthion 20% solution	Follow manufacturer's instructions by wt	Pour on one spot in the middle of the back
	Famophos 13.2% solution	½ fluid oz per 100 lb body wt	Do not exceed 4 fluid oz (120 ml) per animal as the effect may be toxic
	Phosmet 3.8% emulsion	1 fluid oz per 100 lb body wt	Do not exceed 8 fluid oz (240 ml) per animal as the effect may be toxic
	Trichlorfon 8% solution	½ fluid oz per 100 lb body wt	
Spray	Coumaphos 0.375%– 0.5% emulsion		Spray at least 300 lb pressure. Use the 0.5% emulsion when spraying in the northern U.S. or when the animal's hair is long
	Phosmet 0.25% emulsion	1 gallon per adult animal	Spray at high pressure
	Trichlorfon 1% solution	Follow manufacturer's instructions by wt	Spray at at least 300 lb pressure
Dip	Coumaphos 0.25% suspension	Follow manufacturer's instructions	Mix dip well before each use

As soon as the heel fly season is over in your area (consult with your veterinarian or county extension agent) cattle should be treated as soon as possible, but not later than 3 months before the grubs are expected to show up on the animals' backs.

The following chart indicates which insecticides should be used to treat grubs, in which ways, and at what dosages. Pour-on insecticides are measured according to an animal's weight and then poured evenly along the length of its back, making sure that its sides get wet as well. The only exception to this is when using a 20 percent solution of fenthion, which is poured onto only one spot on the back. If you use a spray make sure the animal's skin is good and wet and that the emulsion or solution is well mixed and doesn't separate while being applied. Coumaphos is the only insecticide that should be used as a dip.

Grub Treatment Warnings

The insecticides used to kill cattle grubs are extremely powerful and must be applied strictly in accordance with the manufacturer's instructions. Too much of a good thing with these chemical agents will be fatal to the animals you are treating. Likewise, they are extremely dangerous to other forms of life: human, animal, and plant.

Since these insecticides are absorbed through physical contact and by breathing them, it is necessary to adequately protect yourself when treating cattle for grubs. The following precautions are recommended: a good quality respirator equipped with a filter specifically meant for the insecticide you are using (this should be clearly stated on the package the filter comes in); eye goggles; rubber gloves; rain clothes and changing your clothing often, each time scrubbing yourself well in the shower.

Be sure to apply grub-killing insecticides as soon as the heel fly season in your area ends. Never treat cattle later than 3 months before you estimate the grubs will reach the animals' backs. That is the time they stop migrating and collect in the tissue of the esophagus or the spinal canal, depending on the species. If you were to forget this warning and were to apply an insecticide at this time, the grubs' rapid death in the esophagus would cause a swelling of the throat, problems in swallowing, or a complete inability to do so, drooling, and possible bloat, especially in calves. In a serious case the calf could die of bloat. If the grubs are killed in the spinal canal the calf will be temporarily paralyzed to some degree; in a serious case it could be left permanently paralyzed and would have to be sacrificed.

When treating your cattle isolate them in an area where you can prevent the insecticide from coming in contact with cropland, grazing land, forests, irrigation ditches, rivers or lakes, either as a dust, liquid, or a spray mist. Never mix more than the manufacturer's instructions call for, and only use one systemic insecticide on an animal at any one time. Don't apply these agents on windy days or to animals that have been recently vaccinated, castrated, or operated upon. If they are overheated or are about to be, or have just been shipped, let their grub treatment wait until another day.

Cattle that are being milked or that are nursing calves should not be treated because the insecticide is passed through the milk, constituting a danger to any animal or person that consumes it. Check with your veterinarian to determine how long you should hold recently treated beef and dairy-beef cattle off of the market so that the tiny amount of insecticide that remains in their tissues will not be a health threat if they're processed for meat.

The final word on cattle grubs is that they must be treated for because of the economic loss they represent and the threat they pose to the health of your animals. However, it is necessary to take all of the precautions that are possible to ensure that the treatment isn't worse than the condition caused by the parasites.

Sheep Keds

One of the most common external parasites of sheep and Angora goats is the ked, a blood-sucking fly without wings that spends its whole life living on the animal's body. The female ked gives birth and glues one fully formed larva onto the sheep's wool. This larva is one of 10 white colored, round "eggs" the female will produce in her life, which lasts up to six months. Within 1–2 days, as the larva pupates, it turnes from white to a dark brown. Three weeks later the adult ked emerges from its pupa

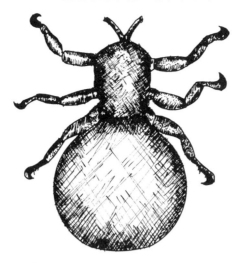

Figure 68. The female sheep ked.

case ready to begin tormenting its host. It is now a quarter-inch long, a reddish-brown color, and covered with short, stiff hairs (see Figure 68).

Sheep keds penetrate the animal's skin with their mouthparts in order to feed by sucking its blood. Yet, unlike ticks, once they have fed they return to the protective environment of the sheep's wool. Because they don't like dusty and very dirty wool, keds are practically never found on the back, preferring instead the shoulders, the sides between the ribs and the hip, the hindquarters, the neck, and the breast.

The spots where keds bite through the skin and feed become irritated, causing sheep to bite at them and rub themselves against posts, fencing, feeders, trees, rocks, or whatever they can find. This attempt to alleviate the itching and discomfort of the bites damages fleeces: they get torn, thinned out, and very dirty. The keds' feces also damage fleeces by permanently staining them, which reduces their value at sale time.

The bites make animals lose strength (in heavy infestations this may be due to anemia) and, in general, cause them to develop poor conditions, especially in young lambs and pregnant ewes. Anytime an animal bites at or rubs its body against a hard object there is a chance it will wound itself. This gives rise to inflammation, further loss of blood, and possible secondary bacterial invasion. Lastly, the time lost from eating during infestations should concern good farm managers.

Oftentimes management practices encourage the spread of sheep keds within a flock. Since keds have no wings they must move from animal to animal via their wool. Thus, when animals are fed, held, or housed in tight areas such as feed lots, nighttime enclosures or winter paddocks keds are able to multiply within flocks.

Sheep Ked Control and Treatment

The best control for keds is shearing. As the fleece is removed so, too, are many adult and pupal keds. Treatment, usually dipping or spraying, but also dusting when you don't want to wet your animals, should be coordinated with shearing.

Right after shearing animals should be completely submerged twice (forced entirely under the surface of the insecticide/water mixture) in a dipping vat containing a powerful insecticide that kills adult keds upon contact and that will leave a strongly concentrated residue on the animal's wool for at least 3-4 weeks. This is a basic requirement of any insecticide you should decide to use because pupating keds are usually protected by their casings during dipping and are only killed once they emerge and come in contact with the chemical residue on the sheep's fleece.

Spraying is also a good way to treat animals; insecticide residues are required for the same length of time as in dipping. Short-haired animals are sprayed at 100-200 pounds per square inch of pressure. Long-haired animals are sprayed with pressures of 300-350 pounds per square inch. Make sure animals are wet to the skin and that the procedure described in "Lice Control and Treatment," p. 88, for horses, mules, donkeys, and cattle is followed.

Recommended Insecticides

The following table of insecticides recommended for use against sheep keds has been adapted from the *Merck Veterinary Manual*, fifth edition, 1979. I have only listed those chemical agents which combine the qualities mentioned previously as necessary to treat animals against sheep keds. All are able to kill adult keds upon contact and leave sufficiently concentrated residue on the sheep's fleece for 3-4 weeks in order to kill keds newly emerging from their pupae cases. Another quality all of these insecticides share is that after you have used them for ked treatment you may send your sheep to market immediately. None of these insecticides build up residues in the animal's tissues necessitating that it be held off of the market for a minimum period to lessen the danger of poisoning in case of human consumption.

Use of the Sheep Ked Insecticide Table

This table is divided into five columns entitled Method of Treatment, Name of Insecticide, What Form is Used, How to Prepare the Mixture, and Other Information. The Method of Treatment is self-explanatory. Under Name of Insecticide you may find one or two chemical agents. If there are two chemicals listed you must buy each one separately and then use them together (in proportions given in How to Prepare the Mixture). In What Form is Used you will find either emulsifiable concentrates or powders. Emulsifiable concentrate means that the insecticide is a concentrated (meaning strong solution) liquid which will form an emulsion when poured into water. The insecticide will literally be suspended in the water without mixing with it. For this reason it is important to keep agitating the water and insecticide to keep the chemical evenly dispersed.

In How to Prepare the Mixture I have given two types of measurements: milliliters (ml), one thousandth of a liter, and teaspoons and tablespoons. A standard teaspoon holds 4 ml and a standard tablespoon hold 15 ml. Measurements in milliliters are exact but not very practical on the farm. Few farmers have the proper equipment to measure in milli-

SHEEP KED INSECTICIDE TABLE

Method of Treatment	Name of Insecticide	What Form Is Used	How to Prepare the Mixture	Other Information
Dip	Dioxathion	Emulsifiable Concentrate	Mix 5.75 ml (1-1½ tsp) Dioxathion with each gallon of water	Dangerous to use more than once in 14 days
	Dioxathion and Dichlorvos	Emulsifiable Concentrate	Mix 57.6 ml (4 tbsp) Dioxathion and 1.9 ml (or ½ tsp) Dichlorvos with each 10 gallons of water	Dangerous to use more than once in 14 days
Spray	Crotoxyphos	Emulsifiable Concentrate	Mix 9.6 ml (2-½ tsp) Crotoxyphos with each gallon of water	Spray on 1 gallon per animal. Dangerous to use more than once in 7 days
	Crotoxyphos and Dichlorvos	Emulsifiable Concentrate	Mix 115 ml (or 7-½ tbsp) Crotoxyphos and 7.7 ml (or 2 tsp) Dichlorvos with each 10 gallons of water	Spray on 1 gallon per animal. Dangerous to use more than once in 14 days
	Dioxathion	Emulsifiable Concentrate	Mix 5.75 ml (or 1-½ tsp) Dioxathion with each gallon of water	Dangerous to use more than once in 14 days
	Dioxathion and Dichlorvos	Emulsifiable Concentrate	Mix 57.6 ml (or 4 tbsp) Dioxathion and 1.9 ml (or ½ tsp) Dichlorvos with each 10 gallons of water	Dangerous to use more than once in 14 days
	Malathion	Emulsifiable Concentrate or Powder	Mix 19.2 ml (or 5 tsp) Malathion with each gallon of water	Don't use on lambs or kids less than 1 month old. Wet animals to the skin
Dust	Malathion	Powder	The powder you use should contain 4–5% Malathion and 95–96% other inert ingredients	Don't use on lambs or kids less than 1 month old
	Malathion and Methoxychlor	Powder	The powder you use should contain 4% Malathion, 5% Methoxychlor, and 91% other inert ingredients	

liters but everyone has a teaspoon and a tablespoon. They fit easily in your pocket and you can carry them to wherever you're dipping, spraying, or dusting. However, one word of caution: both teaspoon and tablespoon measurements are approximate.

I have given you the teaspoon and tablespoon measurements that come as close to the exact milliliter figures as possible and that are practical to use. One teaspoon or tablespoon means all the spoon will hold without overflowing. Adhere strictly to the recommendations in How to Prepare the Mixture. Don't make the mistake of measuring carelessly or of adding a little bit more to really make sure you kill those keds once and for all. All of the recommended insecticides are powerful chemicals. If they are used incorrectly, both your animals' health and your earnings will suffer.

The Sheep Nose Bot Fly

The sheep nose bot fly is gray-brown, covered with short, stiff hairs, and is a little larger than the housefly (see Figure 69). It is named for the part of the sheep's body where the female deposits her young larvae, and may also be known as the sheep gadfly or nasal fly. This parasite occurs throughout the world and may attack goats as well as sheep, although this happens infrequently.

Adult sheep bot flies may live from a few days to 2 weeks, depending on the weather, after emerging from their pupal casings. They mate and the female attacks sheep over and over again in order to deposit up to 500 tiny white larvae in and around their nostrils. Adult flies don't bite, suck blood, or feed at all, but die as soon as depositing all their eggs. They fly very quickly and terrorize animals by hovering in front of their faces and by darting in and around their noses, though they never land on them.

Once the young larvae have been deposited on the nostrils they crawl into the nasal passages and onto the mucous membranes where they feed on the mucus secreted by the nasal tissue. At this stage the larvae are one-sixteenth inch long, very thin, and have practically no color. They crawl far enough into the nasal passages so that they are secure despite the sheep's attempts to dislodge them and expel them by sneezing.

These tiny larvae molt and are transformed into more mature second-stage larvae that are whiter, a little fatter, and that now measure three-sixteenths inch. They continue crawling further into the nasal cavity until they reach the sinuses. Here the larvae molt again. At first they are cream colored, but quickly turn dark as they grow. Fully grown larvae are 1 inch long and a quarter-inch in width, with black bands on their backs (see Figure 70).

The mature larvae begin to crawl from the head cavity back to the nostrils. As they migrate they feed on the mucus which is now heavily secreted by the nasal tissue in response to the irritation caused by their hooked mouthparts and the sharp, spinelike hairs on the undersides of their bodies. Reaching the nostrils, the larvae fall to the ground and burrow under the surface. Here, a few inches underground, they spend 21-63 days pupating before emerging as adult flies. The flies mate and the cycle begins again.

In warm weather and in regions with mild winters this life cycle continues throughout the year. Immature larvae are continuously deposited

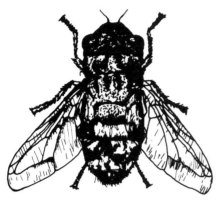

Figure 69. The sheep nose bot fly.

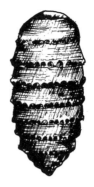

Figure 70. A mature nose bot larva.

on the nostrils by female flies that have emerged from their pupal cases and mated. These first-stage larvae molt and crawl to the sinuses where they replace fully grown larvae returning to the nostrils. The second-stage larvae molt again and mature. Then they too migrate back to the nostrils, fall to the ground, pupate, and develop into sheep nose bot flies.

The only exception to this process is in areas where winters are cold. During the first hard freeze flies and mature, pupating larvae in the ground are killed. However, in a unique response to this climatic threat, bot flies have evolved a survival technique: the first-stage, immature larvae in the nasal passages remain dormant (inactive) from the beginning of cold fall weather until the arrival of spring. Then they once again begin their migration and growth. This explains why, in warm climates, the larval cycle can take as little as a month and in cold climates 10 times longer.

Signs of Attack and Infestation

Sheep become nervous and alarmed when attacked by bot flies. They stop grazing peacefully and run about wildly, with their noses close to the ground, or else they stand still and hold their heads down in order to protect their nostrils. With their heads lowered they appear to be staring intently at the ground and may shake their heads from side to side, sneeze, or stamp their hooves. Since bot flies make their most determined attacks during the hottest part of the day, sheep often group in small circles during this time as a protective measure. They all lower their heads and hold them close together as they face inward.

The most common sign of infestation with bot fly larvae as they crawl through the nasal passages is a flow of clear mucus from the nostrils. When mature larvae move around in the sinuses and return to the nostrils the mucous flow becomes heavier and turns from white-yellow to the green color of pus; it may contain streaks of blood as well. These thick mucous flows from the nostrils are sometimes called *snotty nose*. Healthy sheep aren't bothered by the mucus and have no trouble clearing their nasal passages.

In bad infestations the mucous membranes become thicker than normal. When this and heavy mucous flows occur at the same time animals, especially old and sick ones, have difficulty breathing. They may sneeze repeatedly to try and clear their nasal passages. Sometimes, because of

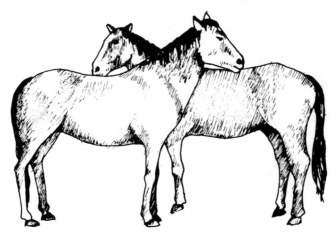

Figure 71.   The typical position of horses protecting themselves from nose bot flies.

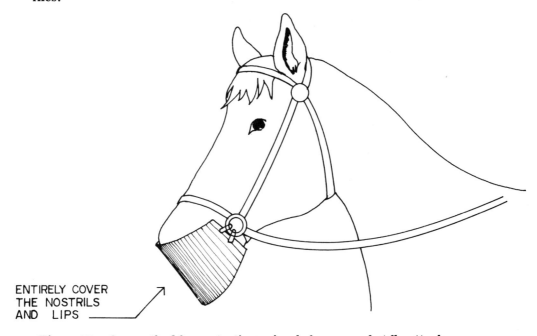

ENTIRELY COVER
THE NOSTRILS
AND LIPS ——————

Figure 72.   One method for protecting animals from nose bot fly attacks.

the thickened mucous membranes, mature larvae can't get out of the sinuses and die there. The sinuses may become inflamed and infected, with abscesses developing. Every once in a while a particularly bad infection spreads to the brain and the animal dies. See Figure 71 for the typical protective position that animals adopt when being attacked.

Treatment

Drench your animals with Ruelene (50 milligrams/pound of body weight) and be sure to follow the manufacturer's instructions, one of the most important of which is that you must wait at least 2 weeks after the treatment before slaughtering. Rafoxanide may also be used, either as a drench or a bolus (3.5 milligrams/pound of body weight).

See Figure 72 for a method to protect animals from nose bot flies.

14

INTERNAL PARASITES

Internal parasites are forms of animal life ranging in size from the one-celled protozoa to 25-foot-long tapeworms that live inside of animals for all or part of their lives. They utilize the animal's body fluids and tissues for their nourishment and development, or in some cases, as a convenient resting place before being consumed by another animal inside of which they continue their life cycle.

The host (animal environment within which an internal parasite feeds, develops, or rests before continuing its maturation process), may be a domestic farm or wild animal, a household pet such as a cat or dog, a bird, an insect, or even a snail. Hosts may be either intermediate or final (also called *definitive*). Intermediate hosts are those in which parasites pass through the various stages of their larval development before reaching their final living place. Final hosts are those in which internal parasites are able to complete their life cycles, attaining maturity, and within which they may reproduce.

Parasites' one-sided relationships with the animals they live in can be very harmful to their hosts, even to the point of killing them, or their presence may cause only a minor disturbance. Whichever the case, the mechanism of their transmission, a familiarity with the signs of infestation, their treatment and control, both natural and chemical, are necessary parts of any effective livestock operation and are discussed in further sections.

The four major kinds of internal parasites that affect livestock are the protozoa, flatworms, roundworms, and thorny-headed worms. Each one deserves a more detailed description.

Protozoa

Protozoa, one-celled, microscopic animals, are among the most primitive forms of life. They are so tiny that it would take 8,000–12,000 of them to make a straight line 1 inch long. Of the four types of protozoa only one, the *sporozoa*, is entirely parasitic; the other three, *flagellatae*, *ciliaphora*, and *rhizopoda* may be either parasitic or free-living—able to provide their own sustenance without need of a host.

The most well-known and widespread sporozoan disease is coccidiosis, which generally attacks young stock, but may affect older animals as well that haven't been exposed to it before or that haven't acquired resistance. Coccidia usually cause an infection that develops very quickly as they attack and begin to destroy the lining of the intestines (and the liver in rabbits). Coccidiosis is a serious, sometimes fatal problem in cattle, sheep, goats, rabbits, and many kinds of birds; it is less serious in horses and pigs. The disease is caused by many factors, but chief among them are stress, overcrowding (especially prevalent in feedlots), and poor sanitary conditions.

The flagellates propel themselves through body fluids with a whiplike motion and are responsible for many blood diseases and reproductive problems throughout the world. The parasitic ciliaphora live in the intestine and move about by vibrating little appendages on the outside of their bodies. The amoebas and rhizopoda, of which there are many varieties, are extremely simple masses of protoplasm (the substance which is the basis of life). They are common parasites in human beings and are found only very rarely in cattle and pigs.

Flatworms

Flatworms are just exactly what their name suggests: flat, soft worms. Two of the most important parasitic members of this group are the flukes and the tapeworms.

Flukes are extremely dangerous worms 1-3 inches long when mature, which may be found in the liver, pancreas, stomach, or blood depending on the type and stage of their development. In each of these locations they attach themselves to tissue with external sucking organs through which they receive thier nourishment. In the case of the disease schistosomiasis, caused by the blood fluke, they attach themselves to the interior of a blood vessel. When flukes are young they may migrate widely through their host's body causing enormous damage to its internal organs and tissues.

The liver fluke, whose intermediate hosts are the snail and black ant, causes one of the most common parasitic diseases in the temperate zones of the world and is responsible for high numbers of sheep and goat deaths, as well as poor health and slow growth of cattle. Its less dramatic but no less important effects are the grading of livers and other meat tissues as unfit for human consumption, damage to internal organs, poor feed conversion, and the general weakening of animal health which may allow infection by secondary invaders (see Figure 73).

Tapeworms in their adult form are long, flat, white, gray, or cream-colored worms. They attach their oval heads to the wall of the intestine and feed themselves through strong, cup-shaped suckers. Their bodies are made up of a series of segments, each one the size of a piece of long-grain rice, which contain both male and female reproductive systems. Usually these segments can be easily seen without magnification.

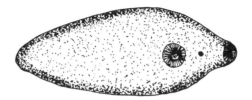

Figure 73.   The liver fluke.

Once tapeworm larvae attach their heads to the intestinal wall it takes them a little more than a month to mature. They are commonly 10 feet in length and at times can measure 25 feet. Having reached maturity they begin to pass eggs and segments of their bodies in the animal's feces. These eggs and segments containing eggs are eaten by insects within which they develop into larvae. In turn the insects are inadvertently eaten or swallowed by livestock grazing on pasture that they or other animals have previously contaminated. Depending on the species, intermediate tapeworm hosts may be beetles, beetle mites, ants, lice, fleas, or grasshoppers. In small numbers tapeworms have a minor effect on an animal's health but in heavy infestations they may cause anemia, digestive upsets, and unthriftiness.

Bladderworms are immature tapeworms whose intermediate hosts are cattle, pigs, sheep, and goats which they parasitize as larvae. Their final hosts may be humans, dogs, or wild canines, such as foxes. Dogs become infested by eating slaughterhouse wastes and animals that die on the range; humans acquire these tapeworms by eating raw or insufficiently cooked meat. Domestic farm animals develop bladderworms by ingesting eggs while grazing on pasture contaminated by either canine or human wastes.

The eggs hatch into larvae in the intestines and then pass through the intestinal walls. The larvae migrate through the body tissues or are carried along by the blood until they reach various internal organs, notably the liver, heart, lungs, and brain. They also attack specialized muscles such as those of the neck and tongue. The degree of damage caused by the different types of bladderworms depends on the number of larvae present, their size, and the particular tissue they destroy. In the case of gid, or staggers, a bladderworm infestation of the brain tissue of sheep and cattle, the animal may lose its coordination and stumble around, as well as lose its appetite and eventually waste away.

Roundworms

Roundworms, also called nematodes, are long, unsegmented, round worms that taper to a tip at each end. They range greatly in size according to the variety, and cause most of the animal diseases associated with parasitic worms.

Roundworms are to be found in practically every part of the body as either migrating larvae or mature adults that have reached their preferred habitat. Larvae occasionally force themselves into tissue or spots in the body they can't get out of. The body responds to these unwelcome intruders by altering the normal structure of its tissue, and wounds and scars result. When an animal is slaughtered these areas are cut out of the edible carcass and declared unfit for human consumption.

Animals are damaged by roundworms in several ways: as the immature worms migrate they force their way through body tissue, disrupting its normal function and injuring it; injured tissue may bleed at a low level for long periods of time causing anemia, or in the case of more serious wounds, hemorrhaging may occur and death result; diarrhea, loss of appetite, stunting of growth in young animals, and loss of weight and condition in animals of all ages are frequently observed. Roundworm infestations often end in the death or permanent injury of the affected host.

In general, the roundworm life cycle is as follows: eggs are passed out in the feces. In a few days to a few weeks, depending on the temperature and humidity, they develop into larvae sandwiched between two protective sheathings which defend them from adverse environmental conditions. Lying in pasture grasses, the larvae are ingested by grazing animals. (Here it's important to mention that some varieties of roundworm larvae, in particular the hookworm and intestinal threadworm, enter the animal by piercing its skin when it lies on dirty bedding or directly on the ground.) Carried along with the grass they reach the digestive tract. Depending on the type of worm, they may settle in the stomach, small intestine, large intestine, or cecum, also called the "blind gut," a small pouch where the large intestine starts. They then emerge from their protective casings. Immature larvae either migrate or remain in their preferred spots. If they don't get trapped or die they develop into mature males and females. After fertilization the female passes her eggs out with the feces and the cycle repeats itself.

Thorny-Headed Worms

Thorny-headed worms are long, pinkish, flat-looking worms that anchor themselves to the wall of the small intestine with their hooked feeding part. This feeding part (for lack of a better term) is not a mouth or a sucker, but merely an opening ringed with six rows of six hoooks each. Since the thorny-headed worm has no digestive system, it absorbs food already digested by its host directly through the host's intestinal wall into its feeding part.

Female worms pass their eggs, containing small larvae, into the feces by the millions. The larvae are protected against the environment by a shell-like layer within which they remain inactive but infective for several years. Once the larval eggs are eaten by their intermediate hosts, white beetle larvae, often called grubs (see Figure 74), they go through

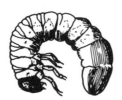

Figure 74.   A white grub.

several stages of development lasting 2–3 months in warm temperatures. Following this they are ready to attack their only final domestic animal host, the pig. Pigs eat white grubs while rooting on pasture or in feedlots. When the grubs reach the pig's digestive tract the larvae emerge and attach themselves to the wall of the small intestine and the cycle is complete.

Thorny-headed worms cause an inflammation of the intestinal wall in pigs. If they should perforate the intestine, peritonitis, an inflammation of the membrane that lines the abdominal cavity and that protects the body's internal organs, usually results, followed by death.

Internal Infestation of Animals

Since the number of parasites that are able to reproduce and subsist from generation to generation within the same host is very small, most internal parasites, in order to survive as species, have evolved life cycles in which they must spend some portion of their lives outside of their final host's bodies. The eggs and larvae which are eliminated by animals in their feces and urine ensure this survival. Yet, adverse environmental conditions kill many eggs and larvae and many more die before reaching their intermediate or final hosts. Because of this natural mortality, mature female parasites produce tremendous amounts of eggs, which are generally covered by protective shells or casings in order to better resist the potentially hostile climates they will encounter.

These eggs and larvae are ingested by many kinds of insects, ants, snails, slugs, and earthworms, which in turn are consumed by livestock as they graze on infected fields or are fed feed that contains parasite-infested manure. Animals may also directly swallow eggs and larvae in soil, water, or feed without them having been eaten by insects or small animals first.

Eggs develop into larvae very quickly in warm weather—generally about a week. These larvae then propel themselves to the upper parts of hay and weeds, moving laboriously along the plants' surface in dry weather and more easily in times of dew, fog, or rain. Once they reach the top of a plant all they need to do is wait for a proper host to come along and give them a free ride to their digestive tract. Likewise, in stables, pens, barns, and anywhere else animals are housed or enclosed, larvae will climb up troughs, doors, gates, fencing, and walls, and onto bedding, litter, and feed. Here they are easily licked off or eaten.

Some larvae gain entrance to their host by biting their way through its skin as it lies on infected bedding, litter, hay, or ground. Other kinds pass through an animal's skin and into its blood as it's being bitten by an insect pest, such as a stablefly or tick. Another all too common method by which parasites are spread is that of eating slaughterhouse waste and dead animals. The flesh and body tissues of the waste and carrion frequently contain infective parasites.

Breeding by natural service, in which a male mounts a female, may also be a means of parasite transmission. Dourine, a flagellate protozoan infection of horses, is spread from one animal to another during copulation and causes death in more than half of the animals affected with it.

Signs of Infestation

Each type of parasite causes its own distinctive effect on the animal species it infests. With experience these signs become apparent indicators of parasitism even in the absence of or low levels of eggs or larvae cultured from a sample of manure. The combination of warm temperatures and high humidity or rain creates the perfect environment for parasite infection. Bear in mind seasonal outbreaks in your region in the past and the physical condition of your animals, and then treat them accordingly.

Should one of your animals die, and if time and expense permit, ask your veterinarian to take a sample of the contents of the digestive tract and a scraping of the lining of the inner wall of its intestines, and examine them under a microscope. This is the best opportunity you'll have to diagnose the health of the rest of your herd and to determine the kinds of parasites they may be harboring.

You must always consider many factors and possibilities before deciding that your animals have parasites, but in general, the following are signs of parasitic infection: circling, stumbling, uncoordinated movements, paralysis, blindness, and drooping eyelids or ears may indicate damage to the central nervous system (the brain and spinal cord). Other symptoms range from loss of appetite and condition, diarrhea, anemia, malnutrition, and hemorrhage to circulatory and respiratory problems, and death. For a specific description of the symptoms of the most important parasites that affect the common farm animals see Chapter 15, The Internal Parasite Guide, p. 130.

Control

Control is a relative term. Ideally, it would be best to eradicate all internal parasites once and for all, yet the most effective means to accomplish that—slaughter of parasite-carrying animals—would put every farmer out of business overnight. So the control we aim for is a more moderate one: keeping parasite numbers in our animals down low enough so that they don't limit the animals' productive ability, and hence our earnings.

There are several ways in which we can accomplish this objective: (a) lower egg and larval infestations of pastures, animal housing, enclosures, and of feeds; (b) treat our animals with antiparasitic drugs on a regular basis and relate this treatment to the animals' developmental stage, climatic conditions, the life cycle of specific parasite invaders, and predictable seasonal outbreaks; (c) indentification of animals that are susceptible to infestation due to age, stage of development or health, (in particular the decrease of immunity to parasite infection following lambing in ewes and the same condition both before and after farrowing in sows); and (d) attempt to develop resistance to infection in our animals.

Point (c) is a particularly crucial and often overlooked step in the control of parasitic infection. Many management faults contribute to an animal's susceptibility to attack—among them are poorly balanced diets, insufficient feed, the overgrazing of pasture, overstocking (too many animals on the same piece of pasture), poor pasture rotation, allowing animals to graze on swampy and marshy land, letting illness and stress conditions go untreated, improper manure disposal, and haphazard parasite control schedules.

Unfortunately, we are frequently our own worst enemies. When we decide to cut back on the mineral supplement because the price is just getting too high and the animals don't really need that much anyway, in spite of what the vet says, or we put the dry cows out on the marshy bottom land in order to save the good pasture for the milkers that are putting milk in the bulk tank and money in our pockets, we often end up costing ourselves much more than the little bit we think we're saving. To those farmers who are fond of telling anyone who'll listen that with market conditions in the shape they are they really can't afford to raise their animals the way they should, the best response I've heard is: "you can't afford not to."

General Control Checklist

1. Don't feed animals directly on the ground.
2. Keep your pastures well drained and animals off of them when they are wet.
3. Don't let your animals graze swampy or marshy land, the edges of ponds, streams, or alongside standing water.
4. Get watering tanks and troughs up off the ground.
5. Prevent your animals from ingesting soil or manure with their feed.
6. Determine optimum stocking levels for each piece of pasture and don't go beyond them.
7. Don't allow overgrazing.
8. If you raise more than one animal species, allow them to graze the same land at different times. By doing so you'll be able to take advantage of their different eating habits (as in the case of cattle, which won't eat the bottom couple of inches of pasture grasses close to the ground unless they are malnourished, and sheep, which closely crop almost everything).
9. Different age groups within the same animal species graze pasture to different heights. Take advantage of this by rotating these different groups through the same pasture, bearing in mind their varying susceptibility to parasite attack. In general, first graze young stock, followed by more resistant adults.
10. Rotate your permanent pastures to reduce parasite egg and larvae numbers.
11. Seeding new temporary pastures each year, if financially feasible, may help reduce continuing parasite problems.
12. Keep young animals separated from older, more parasite resistant stock.
13. Creep feed young cattle, sheep, goats, and pigs before weaning them. This is a method in which unweaned young animals can eat as much grain or specially formulated, balanced feed as they like, while older animals are prevented from doing so.

14. Assume that any new animal added to the herd has parasites. Keep it isolated from the other animals for 3–4 days while you deworm it. Repeat the antiparasite treatment within 3–4 weeks.
15. Develop proper manure treatment practices in order to prevent it from coming in contact with animal feeds and drinking water.
16. Regularly disinfect stables, pens, barns, gates, doors, and housing of all kinds.
17. Change animal bedding and litter once it becomes wet or soiled.
18. Don't allow animals to regularly lie or sleep on dirt that may contain parasite larvae.
19. Bury and lime all the waste products from on-the-farm slaughterings; do the same with any dead animals found on the farm.
20. Keep your dog and cats well wormed. Any strays from off the farm should be kept out.
21. Make sure the sewage system of your house functions properly and don't allow anyone to use the bushes or woods for their bodily functions.
22. Within reason, try to keep imtermediate parasite hosts (snails, slugs, beetles, ants, flies, and so forth) under control.
23. Treat your animals regularly for external parasites.
24. Maintain a regular antiparasitic drug treatment schedule.
25. Develop good all-around management practices and don't sacrifice them for apparent short-term economic advantage. Short cuts in animal health end up costing dearly in the long run.

Different Animals Need Different Controls

Cattle

Dairy cattle suffer frequently from parasitic worms; weaned calves on pasture are the most severely affected age group. They should be kept isolated from the more resistant adults and allowed to graze fields as a group before older animals are turned into it. The calves are moved to a new, ungrazed field before older animals are allowed into the first pasture. Since larvae may remain protected in manure from harsh climatic conditions for several months, merely rotating calf groups through previously grazed pastures would cause them to become infested. Calves must be the first dairy cattle age group let onto any pasture. Some level of immunity to roundworms is developed after two grazing seasons.

Young calves, up to 6 months of age, are especially hard hit by coccidiosis. They acquire the protozoa in stalls, pens, or barns that are dirty with the manure or manure-contaminated litter of older animals or already infected calves. The best control is to not let calves come into contact with the parasite to begin with. This is done by housing calves in their own individual, portable pens until they're big enough (usually when they reach 4–6 months) to turn out into clean pasture.

Beef calves should be creep-fed before weaning in order to strengthen their nutritional levels. The couple of months before and after weaning are those in which they are most vulnerable to parasite attack.

Sheep

Sheep need to be dewormed often, especially during their first year. They never develop very much resistance to parasites and may be reinfected over and over with the same type.

Sheep should be given a broad spectrum dewormer 2 weeks before being bred. They are then moved to pasture that neither they nor any other sheep have grazed on for several months or to fields that have only had cattle on them before. Ewes are dewormed both 1 month before and 1 month after lambing. This is done to combat a decline in resistance after giving birth. Treatment depends on the season, climate, and the normal infective parasites present on the farm and region.

Goats

Goats share many problems in common with sheep. In general, kids are the most severely affected of all age groups, particularly when outbreaks of lung worms, tapeworms, and coccidiosis occur. Good sanitation is important and animals should be kept out of bogs, marshes, swamps, and off of wet land of any type. After deworming goats can be turned into clean pasture after cattle or into root crop fields that haven't previously been grazed.

Pigs

Piglets, like the young of most species, are the most susceptible to parasite attack and injury. They are treated with a broad spectrum, antiparasitic drug when they are 5-6 weeks of age and again a month later. Sows and gilts, young females that haven't had their first litter yet, are dewormed 5-7 days before being bred and before farrowing. They are also dewormed midway through their lactation. Fattening pigs are dewormed at 110 pounds and boars twice a year.

Sows relax their resistance to parasite infection during a period that stretches from 2 weeks before farrowing until 6 weeks afterward. If they are infected with roundworms during their pregnancy and not treated, they pass a large number of eggs in their feces from farrowing up until weaning. If pens aren't kept clean during this period piglets run a high risk of becoming infected.

Pens and housing should always be disinfected before farrowing and again up to a week after each antiparasite treatment. Parasite problems must always be considered threats that affect the whole herd. If you are confronted with a serious parasite outbreak in one group, assume all your animals are affected and treat the whole herd. Sanitation and hygiene are very important and must be checked every day. Any pig introduced into the herd from off the farm must be dewormed before joining its new herdmates.

Poultry

Since poultry are subject to attack by so many varieties of parasitic worms (over 60 in the United States alone) and since the control of poultry parasites is dependent to a large degree on management practices, it is advisable to work closely with your veterinarian to develop a parasite control plan designed specifically for your farm.

Treatment

Internal parasite treatment is generally effected through the use of broad spectrum drugs, those that kill a wide range of harmful organisms. However, antiparasitic drugs are not a cure-all. They help to reduce parasite numbers, but must be used in coordination with the different control measures explored in preceding sections.

Drug use is always aimed at the weakest link in the parasite life cycle. The optimal time to use an antiparasitic drug is when climatic conditions are the harshest and most threatening to the survival of the free-living egg or larval stages of the attacking parasite. Treatment at this point will reduce the contamination of the animal's habitat for a long time.

If the perfect broad spectrum, antiparasitic drug existed, which it doesn't (although several pharmaceutical firms are determined to develop and market it), it would kill eggs, larvae, and mature parasites without injuring the animal's health. It would not remain in the host's blood or tissues for more than a very short time, and would not cause parasites to develop resistance to its effectiveness over several generations (as presently happens with the repeated use of some broad spectrum drugs). It would be possible to administer it in a number of ways— for example, as an intramuscular injection, a pour-on, or as a powder dust. The perfect antiparasite would not limit or alter the effect of other drugs that were used at the same time to treat other conditions. Finally, it would be inexpensive in relation to the benefits it would provide.

Antiparasitic drugs are administered in many ways: by intramuscular injection, through a drench or a pour-on, in the drinking water, and mixed into the feed, as a powder dust, and in mineral, energy, and salt blocks for use in feedlots and on the range. The specific means of administration should be chosen after a consideration of the seriousness of the infestation and the cost and ease of treatment based on your specific management system. Treatment will be most effective if it is coordinated with the natural environmental factors that threaten the survival of the parasites you want to rid your animals of. A few of these factors are hot and dry weather, the need of free-living eggs and larvae to be ingested by intermediate hosts in order to further develop, and for some parasites in the free-living stage, cold, freezing weather.

When treating your animals make sure all their nutritional needs are being met and that they are moved to clean, parasite-free pastures, or if held in confinement housing, that their feed and water are pure and uncontaminated. Don't treat individual animals in a group; it's a waste of time. Assume they're all infected and treat all of them at the same time. This will break the cycle of needless reinfection from animal to animal and will save you a lot of money.

If you notice a poorer than expected response to treatment, especially if you use the same antiparasitic drugs frequently, drug resistance should be suspected. Consult with your veterinarian for alternative drugs and an evaluation of management practices which may be contributing to the problem. Don't simply decide that more is better and keep dosing your animals. Stop treatment and look for the answer to the problem!

15

THE INTERNAL PARASITE GUIDE

The following parasite guide has been prepared with the aim of informing readers about the specific internal parasites that affect their animals. I feel that it is important for farmers and animal owners to have more information available to them than is usually provided in most veterinary guides that are written for laypeople, yet explained in everyday terms and not in the overly complicated scientific language or jargon which is so often used.

Several facts will emerge from a reading of this guide:

1. Each animal species is attacked by many different kinds of internal parasites.
2. The symptoms of parasite infestations are similar in many cases.
3. Drug treatment is different and specific for the overwhelming majority of parasites and often varies among species of animals when attacked by the same parasite.
4. Many of the causes of parasite infestations and the controls of them are connected with management practices.
5. Recognition of parasite attack and its control and treatment are complicated matters that require a team effort between you, the farmer or animal owner, your veterinarian, and the laboratory you will use to culture the fecal samples you collect.

This guide should not be used as a replacement for your veterinarian; that would almost assuredly be a costly and tragic mistake. It is my hope that with the greater understanding of the complexity of parasite infection that you can gain from a careful examination of this section you will be better able to work together with your veterinarian in the quick recognition of infection, the collection of fecal samples, and the evaluation and design of improved management practices that will assist in the realization of the goal of internal parasite control.

The guide is presented in the form of a table with the following column headings: Animal Species, Common and Scientific Name, Part of the Body Injured, Symptoms, Control and Treatment, and Other Information. Animal Species and Part of the Body Injured are both self-explanatory. The common name refers to the everyday name or names that a parasite is known by. In those cases when there is no common name for a parasite but the disease it causes is well known, I have used the name of the disease before the scientific name. An example of this is coccidiosis. The scientific name is the Latin name assigned to a parasite. I have included it because oftentimes other veterinary guides, the laboratories that analyze the fecal samples you collect, and the antiparasitical drugs you buy use the scientific name rather than the common one. The scientific name appears in parentheses. Symptoms comprise a complicated category. I have listed most of the symptoms that are seen with each different kind of parasite. That doesn't mean they all will be seen or even that any of them will be. One symptom on the list may be observed or several in combination or succession. In general, symptoms are notoriously inaccurate indicators of what parasites infest your animals. Their value lies in enabling you to recognize that your animals are being attacked. Based on that recognition you need to collect and send off feces, urine, or blood samples for laboratory analysis, consult with your veterinarian as to treatment and control, and with his or her help examine the management practices you employ that may be contributing to parasite infection.

The column on Control and Treatment offers suggestions on management changes to treat against and prevent infection. It also lists specific drugs, the ways they should be administered, and at what dosages in order to both treat and prevent parasite attacks. Dosages are given in milligrams per pound of body weight (mg/lb body wt), ounces per pound of body weight, milliliters per pound of body weight (ml/lb body wt), grams per pound of body weight (gm/lb body wt), or milligrams per pound of feed. Drugs are mixed into feed by weighing out the dosage for all the animals you wish to treat and then mixing this quantity thoroughly with a small amount of feed, either by hand or in a mill. This is called a premixture. The premixture is then mixed thoroughly into the total amount of feed that will be given to the animals you will treat. It is tremendously important to completely and evenly distribute the drug throughout the premixture and to then do the same with the premixture in the rest of the ration. Failure to do so may result in the permanent damage or death of your animals through an overdose of one of the very powerful drugs used for treatment. Your veterinarian is the best source of information as to which drug is giving the best results in your area. Always consult with him or her before treating your animals.

The column headed Other Information includes such facts as the climatic and regional distribution of parasites, what their intermediate or final hosts are, their size, color, or shape, their resistance to drug treatment, and how they enter the animal.

Animal Species	Common Name (Scientific Name)	Part of the Body Injured	Symptoms	Control and Treatment	Other Information
Cow	1. Large stomach worm; wire worm; barber pole worm (*Haemonchus Placei*)	Stomach	a. Anemia b. Off and on constipation c. "Bottle jaw" d. Loss of appetite e. Rough hair coat f. Loss of weight g. Weakness h. Death	a. Any of the following drugs may be used for treatment: 1. Oxfendazole given orally (2 mg/lb body wt) 2. Albendazole given orally (3.4 mg/lb body wt) 3. Levamisole given as a drench mixed into the drinking water or as a pour-on (2–5 mg/lb body wt) 4. Thiophanate given as a drench or mixed into the feed (22–45 mg/lb body weight)	a. Occurs mostly in the tropics b. Adult male worms are $7/10''$ long; adult females are $1\text{-}1/5''$ long c. Watch for drug resistance
	2. Medium stomach worm; brown stomach worm (*Ostertagia Ostertagi*)	Stomach	a. A lot of watery diarrhea b. Loss of appetite c. Rough hair coat d. Loss of weight e. Weakness f. Death	a. The same treatment as above	a. Occurs mostly in Temperate Zone regions b. Adult worms are $1/4''\text{–}1/3''$ long c. Adult worms are killed with insecticides; larval stages are often drug resistant d. Watch for drug resistance
	3. Small stomach worm; small hairworm (*Trichostrongylus*	Stomach	a. A lot of watery diarrhea b. Loss of appetite c. Rough hair coat	a. The same treatment as above	a. Adult worms are $1/5''$ long

Parasite	Location	Symptoms	Treatment	Characteristics
axel)		d. Loss of weight e. Weakness f. Death		
4. Intestinal threadworm (*Strongyloides papillosus*)	Small intestine	a. Off and on diarrhea b. Loss of appetite c. Loss of weight d. Blood and mucus in the feces	a. The same treatment as above	a. Threadworm larvae or adults are swallowed or penetrate the skin' b. Only the females are parasitic c. Adult females measure 1/10"–1/4" d. Symptoms aren't often seen
5. Roundworm (*Toxocara vitulorum*)	Small intestine and various organs		a. The same treatment as above	a. Calves are infected through the colostrum b. Calves up to 6 months are attacked; older ones are resistant c. Eggs with pitted shells are seen in the feces d. Adult worms are 8"–12" long, fat and white
6. (*Nematodirus helvetianus*)	Intestines	a. Diarrhea b. Loss of appetite	a. The same treatment as above	a. Adult males are 1/2" long; adult females are 7/10"–1" in length b. Eggs build up in pastures and hatch in great numbers after a rain. They survive from year to year c. Cattle become immune quickly
7. (*Cooperia punctata;*	Small intestine	a. A lot of diarrhea b. Loss of appetite	a. The same treatment as above	a. Adult worms are red, coiled and 1/5"–1/3" long

Animal Species	Common Name (Scientific Name)	Part of the Body Injured	Symptoms	Control and Treatment	Other Information
	Cooperia pectinata; Cooperia oncophora)		c. Wasting away		
	8. Hookworm *(Bunostomum phlebotomum)*	Small intestine	a. Stamping and uneasiness of stabled cattle b. Anemia c. Rapid weight loss d. Alternating diarrhea and constipation	a. The same treatment as above	a. Adult males are 1/3" long; adult females are 7/10" in length b. Hookworm larvae are swallowed or penetrate the skin c. Stabled cattle stamp their hooves and act uneasily as hookworms bite through the skin of their legs d. Penetration of the skin in resistant calves causes surface wounds, pus, and scabs
	9. Large-mouth bowel worm *(Chabertia ovina)*	Small intestine; colon	a. Feces are covered with mucus	a. The same treatment as above	a. Adult worms are 1/2" long
	10. Nodular worm *(Oesophagosto-mum radiatum*	Intestines	a. Loss of appetite b. Serious diarrhea (dark and foul smelling) c. Loss of weight d. Death	a. The same treatment as above	a. Adult worms are 1/2"–3/5" long. b. Adult animals develop nodules in the intestine which reduce movement within it
	11. Tapeworm *(Moniezia expansa; Moniezia*	Not thought to harm animals	a. Tapeworm segments are seen in the feces	a. Any of the following drugs may be used for treatment: 1. Lead arsenate given	a. The intermediate host is a mite b. These tapeworm varieties affect young

	Location	Damage	Control/Treatment	Description
benedeni)			orally (1 g for calves; 2 g for adults), with castor oil given afterwards. 2. Niclosamide given as a drench (22 mg/lb body wt) 3. Albendazole given orally (3.4 mg/lb body wt)	cattle
12. Common liver fluke (*Fasciola hepatica*)	Intestines; liver; bile duct; lungs	a. Enlargement and hemorrhage of the liver b. Enlarged bile duct	a. Prevent access to areas where snails are found b. Control snails by draining wet land or by responsible pesticide use c. Rafoxanide, Brotianide, or Nitroxynil may be used for treatment in the winter d. Check with your vet for the drug recommended for use in your region	a. This fluke is shaped like a leaf, and is 1-1/5" long and 1/2" wide b. The intermediate host is a snail
13. Giant liver fluke (*Fasciola gigantica*)	Intestine: liver; bile duct; lungs	a. The same as with the common liver fluke	a. The same as with the common liver fluke	a. It looks like the common liver fluke but is twice as long (3" when adult) b. It is found in warmer regions than the common liver fluke c. Also affects buffalo
14. Large liver fluke (*Fascioloides magna*)	Liver	a. The liver is badly damaged.	a. Fence deer out of cattle pastures b. Keep cattle off of	a. Adults are 3" long and oval-shaped b. Snails are the in-

Animal Species	Common Name (Scientific Name)	Part of the Body Injured	Symptoms	Control and Treatment	Other Information
				swampy, wet ground where snails are found c. Control snails by draining wet land or by using a pesticide that won't harm other animal species d. Use Rafoxanide for treatment according to the manufacturer's instructions	termediate host; deer are the final one c. If cattle and deer graze close together the cattle are probably infested
	15. Lancet fluke; Lesser liver fluke *Dicrocoelium pendriticum*	Liver; bile duct	a. The liver is badly damaged b. The bile duct is enlarged c. In heavy infestations the cow will have jaundice	a. Keep cattle off of swampy, wet land where snails are found b. Control snails by draining wet land or by using a pesticide that won't harm other animal species c. Several drugs can be used, including Hetolin, Praziquantel, and thiabendazole. Follow manufacturer's instructions	a. Adults are ½" long and thin b. This fluke's first intermediate host is a snail; the second is an ant
	16. Pancreatic fluke (*Eurytrema pancreaticum; E. ovis; E. coelomaticum*)	Pancreatic duct; sometimes the bile duct	a. The pancreatic duct is swollen and may be badly damaged	a. Use Praziquantel or a benzimidazole following the manufacturer's instructions. b. Consult with your vet for control measures and for the recommended drug for use in your region	a. The adult is ⅗" long and ¼" wide b. This fluke is widely distributed in Asia and Brazil c. The first intermediate host is a snail; the second is a grasshopper

136

#	Parasite	Location	Signs	Treatment / Control	Description
17.	Stomach fluke (There are many species)	Small intestine; rumen (the first stomach); reticulum (the second stomach)	Fluke larvae cause: a. Bad inflammation of the small intestine b. Loss of appetite c. Tremendous thirst d. Bad diarrhea e. Death (especially in young animals)	a. Keep cattle off of wet and swampy land where they may ingest snails b. Control snails as explained above c. Use Resorantel according to the manufacturer's instructions	a. Adults are 3/5" long, pink or red, and look like tiny pears b. The intermediate host is a snail
18.	Blood fluke (caused by many species of schistosomes)	Liver; the intestines; blood vessels; lungs; bladder; pancreas; the nasal passages	a. Blood flukes of the intestines and liver: 1. Anemia 2. Inflammation and hemorrhage of the intestines 3. Wasting away 4. Death b. Blood flukes of the nasal passages: (Seen in bad infestations) 1. A lot of mucus flows from the nostrils 2. Snoring 3. Difficulty in breathing	a. Keep cattle off of wet and swampy land. b. Control snails as explained above c. Use Trichlorfon, hydrochloride hycanthone, lucanthone, or Stibophen under the direction of your vet.	a. Adults are very thin, 1 1/5" long and are found in blood cells b. This fluke is found in some countries along the Mediterranean Sea, in Africa, Asia, the Middle East, and the Carribean. c. The intermediate host is an aquatic snail d. There are three major kinds: blood flukes of the intestines, liver, and nose.
19.	Lungworm (Dictyocaulus viviparus)	Lungs	a. Coughing b. Fast, short breathing c. The head is extended forward with the mouth open and drooling d. Loss of appetite	a. Calves should be isolated from adults with lungworms and kept off of pasture where they have grazed b. Vaccination c. Drench with Levamisole	a. Occurs in Temperate Zone areas with high humidity throughout the world. b. Usually affects young cattle during the first year on pasture.

Animal Species	Common Name (Scientific Name)	Part of the Body Injured	Symptoms	Control and Treatment	Other Information
			e. Wasting away f. Sudden fall off in milk production g. Lungs fill with fluid	or mix it in the drinking water (2–5 mg/lb of body wt) d. Give Oxfendazole orally (2 mg/lb of body wt) e. Give Albendazole orally (3.4 mg/lb of body wt) f. Give Cambendazole as a bolus, a very large pill, (11.5 mg/lb of body wt) g. Give Fenbendazole orally (3.4 mg/lb of body wt)	c. Lungworm attacks last about 3 months. Surviving animals have a strong immunity d. After deworming put cattle on clean pasture and feed them well
	20. Stephanofilariasis (*Stephanofilaria stilesi*)	The skin between the brisket and the abdomen	a. The skin becomes inflamed between the brisket and the abdomen b. The skin may be covered with bloody wounds or be dry, smooth, and have lost its hair	There is presently no known treatment for stephanofilariasis other than control of the horn fly to prevent infection.	a. Adult worms are $\frac{1}{10}$″–$\frac{1}{5}$″ long and lie just below the surface of the skin b. The intermediate host is the female horn fly c. The parasite is found all through the U.S., but is most common in the West and Southwest
	21. Coccidiosis (*Eimeria zuernii; E. Bovis; E. ellipsoidalis; E. auburnensis*)	Small intestine Large intestine	a. Mild infection: 1. Watery manure b. Serious infection: 1. Watery diarrhea containing blood or mucus 2. Loss of appetite 3. Weight loss 4. Dehydration 5. Depression	a. Proper sanitation b. Good nutrition and fresh, clean water c. Reduce stress conditions d. Any of the following drugs can be used for treatment: 1. Give sulfaquinoxaline orally 3–5 days	a. Generally affects 1-month-old calves to 1-year-old cows b. Older cattle are usually resistant but may infect younger animals. Secondary infections, like pneumonia, may occur c. Occurs off and on

No.	Disease (organism)	Organs affected	Symptoms	Treatment/Control	Remarks
			6. Trying to urinate or defecate without being able to 7. Death	(6 mg/lb body wt daily) 2. Give sulfamerazine sodium orally (60 mg/lb body wt. Follow with 30 mg/lb of body wt each 24 hrs during 4 days) 3. Give sulfamethazine orally or IV (100 mg/lb body wt the first day. Follow this with 50 mg/lb body wt once each day for 3–4 days). e. For preventive treatment of calves mix Amprolium daily into the feed or drinking water (225 mg/100 lbs body wt each day for 21 days)	during rainy seasons and frequently in feed lots in cold weather d. Treat healthy animals preventively when coccidiosis cases occur in feed lots or on pasture e. It's important to prevent dehydration
22.	(Besnoitia besnoiti)	Skin; blood vessels; mucus membranes	a. Fever b. Loss of appetite c. Fear of and avoidance of light d. The skin thickens, wrinkles, and becomes hard e. Inflammation of the nose and its mucous membrane f. Movement causes pain g. Hair and skin fall off	a. Vaccination with a live vaccine (only done in a few countries) b. Isolate affected animals c. Check with your vet for recommended drug treatment	a. Besnoitiosis is caused by protozoan parasite b. The definitive host is the cat c. Badly infected bulls usually become sterile d. Cattle that have been infected are carriers of the parasite as long as they live

Animal Species	Common Name (Scientific Name)	Part of the Body Injured	Symptoms	Control and Treatment	Other Information
	23. (Sarcocystis cruzi; S. hominis; S. tenella)	Muscles; tissue lining the heart and blood vessels; nerve tissue	h. Wasting away a. In mild infections there are no symptoms b. In serious infections: 1. Fever 2. Loss of appetite 3. Drop in milk production 4. Diarrhea 5. Anemia 6. Spasms 7. Wasting away 8. Weakness 9. Abortion 10. Collapse 11. Death	a. Don't let dogs or cats eat dead cattle or slaughter wastes b. Keep dogs and cats off of cattle pasture, out of cattle housing, and out of feed mills and grain storage areas c. For a preventative treatment feed Amprolium daily for 30 days (45 mg/lb body wt daily) d. For drug treatment in case of serious infection check with your vet	a. Sarcosystosis is a protozoan disease b. The cow is an intermediate host which is eaten by a final host (either a cat, dog, or human) in order to complete this protozoan's life cycle c. Cattle become infected by swallowing spores on pasture or in feed that are voided in dog, cat, or human feces
Horses	1. Common bot (Gasterophilus intestinalis)	Mouth; stomach	a. Inflammation of the mouth b. It may be painful for the horse to eat	1 month after the first hard frost give Dichlorvos once in the feed (14–19 mg/lb of body wt) or a 12.3% solution of Triclorfon with a stomach tube (½ fluid oz/100 lb body wt)	a. The parasite that causes this infestation is the larva of the horse botfly b. Eggs are laid on hair all over the body, but particularly on the front legs and shoulders c. Since eggs are laid in the summer, assume that your animals are infected each fall
	2. Nose or lip bot (Gasterophilus haemorrhoidalis)	Mouth; stomach	Same as with the common bot	Same as with the common bot	The eggs are laid on the hairs of the lips

	Location	Symptoms	Treatment	Remarks
3. Throat bot (*Gasterophilus nasalis*)	Mouth; small intestine	Same as with the common bot	Same as with the common bot	The eggs are laid on the hairs of the lower jaw
4. (*Draschia megastoma*)	Stomach; peritoneum	a. Upset stomach b. Poor digestion c. Sharp pain in the belly or bowels d. Stomach tumors e. Inflammation of the membrane lining the abdominal cavity f. Death	a. Control house and stable flies b. Carbon disulfide given orally (2 ml/100 lbs of body wt, *but don't ever give more than 20 ml*) will kill parasites in the body cavity but won't have any effect on those in the stomach wall	a. House and stable flies are the intermediate hosts b. The flies or the parasite larvae they carry are swallowed as the flies feed on the horses' lips
5. Small stomach worm (*Trichostrongylus axei*)	Stomach	a. Inflammation of the stomach lining b. A lot of mucus is produced	a. Thiabendazole in a huge dosage is the only known drug treatment b. Check with your vet	a. Mature worms are ⅓" long and very thin
6. (*Parascaris equorum*)	The intestines	a. Generally poor condition b. Diarrhea c. No energy d. Sometimes a sharp pain in the belly or bowels	Give Thiabendazole—Piperazine Phosphate, also called Equizole A, orally (1½ oz/500 lb body wt) or any broad spectrum antiparasite used for horses	a. All adult worms are 1⅕" long and fat b. Foals are most heavily affected
7. Bloodworm; Palisade worm; Red worm (*Strongylus vulgaris; S. Edentatus; S. Equinus*)	Arteries; small and large intestines; liver; pancreas; testicles	a. Anemia b. Weakness c. Diarrhea d. Wasting away e. Sharp pain in the belly f. Inflammation of the intestines	a. Use Thiabendazole (200 mg/lb body wt) or a large dose of Fenbendazole against larvae b. Mature worms are treated for every 6 to 8 weeks with:	a. It should be assumed that horses on pasture are infected and should be treated regularly b. These worms migrate a lot through the body c. Dichlorvos may cause sharp pains in the belly or bowels

Animal Species	Common Name (Scientific Name)	Part of the Body Injured	Symptoms	Control and Treatment	Other Information
	8. Pinworm (Oxyuris equi)	Large intestine; rectum	a. Yellowish crust around the anus b. Itching and rubbing of the tail and anus	1. Dichlorvos, once in the feed, (14–19 mg/lb body wt) 2. Pyrantel or Tartrate, also in the feed (5 g/100 lb body wt)	a. Adult females are 1/3"–3/5" long; males are smaller. b. Because of itching, horses will rub off the hair in spots on their rump and break the hairs of the tail
	9. (Strongyloides Westeri)	Small intestine	a. Diarrhea in foals	Use Dichlorvos, Pyrantel, Fenbendazole, or Thiabendazole according to the manufacturer's instructions	
	10. Tapeworm (Anoplocephala magna)	Small intestine; stomach	In bad infections there may be anemia and digestive upsets	a. Use Thiabendazole orally (20 mg/lb body wt) or b. Cambendazole as a bolus (9 mg/lb body wt)	a. Adults are 1" long b. Eggs are seen in the manure
	11. Tapeworm (Anoplocephala perfoliata)	Small intestine; cecum	Same as above	Treat with Niclosamide or Dichlorophen according to the manufacturer's instructions	Eggs are seen in the manure
	12. Tapeworm (Paranoplocephala mamillana)	Small intestine; stomach	Same as above	Same as above	a. Adults are 1/3" long b. Eggs are seen in the manure
	13. Lungworm	Lungs	a. Deep cough	Check with your vet as to	a. Common throughout

	Organ affected	Signs	Treatment	Notes
(Dictyocaulus arnfieldi)			which of the benzi-midazoles to use	the world b. Also affects donkeys c. Occurs in temperate areas with high humidity d. Usually affects young horses during their first year on pasture
14. (Besnoitia bennetti)	Skin; blood vessels; mucous membranes	a. Fever b. Loss of appetite c. Fear of and avoidance of light d. The skin thickens, wrinkles and becomes hard e. Inflammation of the nose and its mucous membrane. f. It hurts to move. g. Hair and skin fall off h. Wasting away	a. Isolate affected animals b. Check with your vet for recommended drug treatment	a. Besnoitiosis is caused by a protozoan parasite b. The definitive host is the cat c. Horses that have been infected are carriers of the parasite as long as they live
Pigs				
1. Red stomach worm (Hyostrongylus rubidus)	Stomach	*In heavy infestations:* a. Intermittant changes in appetite b. Anemia c. Diarrhea d. Drop in normal weight e. Inflammation of the stomach wall with a lot of mucus produced f. Occasional hemorrhage of the stomach	a. Feed a paste of Thiabendazole (30–40 mg/lb body wt) or b. Give Levamisole as a drench, in the drinking water or as a bolus (2–5 mg/lb body wt)	a. Adults are ¼″ long and very thin b. Most common in pigs on pasture

Animal Species	Common Name (Scientific Name)	Part of the Body Injured	Symptoms	Control and Treatment	Other Information
	2. Thick stomach worm (*Ascarops Strongylina; Physocephalus sexalatus*)	Stomach	wall leading to death *In heavy infestations:* a. Intermittant changes in appetite b. Anemia c. Diarrhea d. Drop in normal weight	a. After not feeding pigs for 36 hours give carbon disulfide orally in capsules or via a stomach tube (8–10 ml/100 lbs body wt) or b. A Piperazine–carbon disulfide complex, also called Parvex, mixed into ¼ of the normal amount of feed the animal consumes per day (60 mg/lb body wt)	a. Adults are ½" long and fatter than the red stomach worm b. Most common in pigs on pasture c. The intermediate host is a manure-eating beetle.
	3. Large round worm (*Ascaris suum*)	Small intestine; bile duct; stomach; liver; lungs	a. Weight loss b. Poor condition and growth c. Stunting of young animals d. Possible blockage and rupture of intestine e. Possible blockage of bile duct causing jaundice f. Hemorrhage of the liver g. Swelling of the lungs with fluid. This causes a thumping sound as the pig breathes	a. Migrating immature worms are treated with Pyrantel Tartrate mixed into the feed (10 mg/lb body wt) b. For adult worms use any of the following: 1. Piperazine orally (50 mg/lb body wt) 1. Cambendazole as a paste, bolus, or in the feed (1 mg/lb body wt) 3. Fenbendazole orally (4.6 mg/lb body wt) 4. Pyrantrel Tartrate mixed in the feed (10 mg/lb body wt) 5. Levamisole as a	a. Adults are 1⅕" long and fat b. Young pigs up to 4–5 months are the most severely affected c. Blockage of bile duct, causing jaundice, by adult worms is common in pigs that haven't been fed for some time while being transported to market d. If the lungs are affected infection by secondary bacterial invaders is probable and must be treated for e. Roundworm eggs are killed in a few weeks by

144

Parasite	Location	Signs/Damage	Treatment and Control	Characteristics
4. Intestinal threadworm (*Strongyloides ransomi*)	Small intestine	In heavy infestations: a. Anemia b. Diarrhea c. Wasting away d. Death	drench, a bolus, or mixed in the feed or the drinking water (2–5 mg lb body wt) a. To treat adult worms use either of the following: 1. Thiabendazole orally as a paste (30–40 mg/lb body wt) 2. Cambendazole orally as a paste or bolus or mixed into the feed or drinking water (9 mg/lb body wt) b. To limit infection of piglets via the colostrum give Mebendazole to the sow in her feed for a few days before and after farrowing	direct sunlight and very dry conditions a. Of the adults only the female is parasitic b. Baby pigs are infected by eggs passed in the colostrum
5. Thorny-headed worm (*Macracanthorhynchus hirudinaceus*)	Small intestine	a. Part of the intestine that the worm attaches itself to is inflamed b. Destruction of parts of the intestinal wall c. Possible inflammation of the membrane that surrounds the abdomen, leading to death	a. Disinfect pens b. Keep pigs off infected pastures c. Give Levamisole as a drench, a bolus, or mixed into the feed or drinking water (2–5 mg/lb body wt)	a. Adults males are 2/5" long; females are up to 2 3/5". Both are flat b. Several kinds of beetles act as the intermediate host

Animal Species	Common Name (Scientific Name)	Part of the Body Injured	Symptoms	Control and Treatment	Other Information
	6. Nodular worm (Oesophagostomum dentatum)	Large intestine	In heavy infestations (however, these signs may be caused by secondary invaders): a. Thickening of the wall of the large intestine b. Loss of appetite c. Digestive upsets d. Wasting away	a. Use any of the following drugs for treatment: 1. Give Levamisole orally as a drench, bolus, or mixed into the feed or drinking water (2–5 mg/lb body wt) 2. Piperazine hexahydrate mixed into the drinking water of growing pigs after not letting them drink for 24 hrs (50 mg/lb body wt) 3. Give Piperazine salts orally to mature pigs (50 mg/lb body wt) 4. Mix Pyrantel tartrate into the feed (10 mg/lb body wt)	a. Adult worms are $1/3$″ long, very thin and white colored b. More eggs are produced around farrowing and during lactation than normally c. Pigs become directly infected while feeding on contaminated ground or pasture d. Intermediate hosts are a fly or various rodents e. Pigs 3 months and older are most susceptible
	7. Whipworm (Trichuris suis)	Small and large intestines	a. Loss of appetite b. Anemia c. Difficulty breathing d. Diarrhea e. Poor growth f. Wounds in the intestinal wall g. Uncoordinated movements h. Wasting away i. Death	a. Use Levamisole orally as a drench, a bolus, or mixed in the feed or drinking water (2–5 mg/lb body wt) or b. Give Fenbendazole or Oxfendazole after consulting with your veterinarian	a. Adults are $1/10$″–$1/3$″ long b. In a heavy infestation the pig will be attacked by secondary bacterial invaders
	8. B. coli	Large intestine	In young pigs: a. Anemia	a. Good sanitation	a. B. coli is a microscopic ciliate protozoan

Parasite	Organs Affected	Symptoms	Treatment/Control	Facts
(Balantidium coli)		b. Slower than normal growth c. Inflammation of the intestines	b. Consult with your vet for drug treatment	b. Baby pigs are infected by eating the sow's feces c. Can be transmitted to humans

9. Trichinella (Trichinella spiralis)	Intestines stomach; most muscles; heart; central nervous system	In heavy infestations intestinal symptoms occur first, followed by muscular symptoms:
		a. Intestinal symptoms:
		  1. Diarrhea
		  2. Low fever
		  3. Abdominal pain
		  4. Nausea
		  5. Vomiting
		b. Muscular symptoms:
		  1. Loss of appetite
		  2. Muscles are stiff, swollen, hard and painful
		  3. Difficulty in breathing
		  4. Low fever
		  5. Wasting away
		  6. Occasional death
			a. Cook all garbage fed to pigs at 212°F for 30 minutes
			b. Institute a thorough rodent control program on your farm.
			c. Good sanitation
			d. Once pigs are infected consult with your vet as to how to reduce the pain they are in until they either die or survive
				a. This nematode causes a serious disease in humans, most commonly in the Temperate and Arctic zones, called trichinosis that is constracted by eating undercooked pork
				b. Adults are $1/20''$–$3/20''$ long
				c. Pigs infect each other by passing larvae in the feces

10. Lungworm (Metastrongylus elongatus)	Small intestine; heart; lungs	a. Pigs less than 6 months old that are heavily infected:
		  1. Loss of appetite
		  2. Poor condition
		  3. Weight loss
		  4. Coughing
		  5. Difficulty breathing
			Any of the following drugs can be used:
			a. Levamisole orally as a drench or a bolus, or mixed into the feed or drinking water (2–5 mg/lb of body wt)
			b. Cambendazole orally as a paste or bolus or mixed into the feed (9
				a. This parasite occurs throughout the world
				b. Its intermediate hosts are most kinds of earthworms
				c. Adult males are 1" long; females are almost 2". Both worms are thin and white
				d. Pigs older than 6

Animal Species	Common Name (Scientific Name)	Part of the Body Injured	Symptoms	Control and Treatment	Other Information
				mg/lb body wt) c. Give Fenbendazole orally (2.3 mg/lb body wt) d. Administer Oxfendazole or Albendazole after checking with your vet as to the dosage	months are usually immune
	11. Common liver fluke (*Fasciola hepatica*)	Intestine; liver; bile duct	Usually there are none	a. Don't let pigs pasture on land that has been grazed by sheep or cattle b. Keep pigs off marshy and swampy land and wet spots where snails are to be found	a. Sheep and cattle are the normal final hosts but pigs occasionally become infected b. The intermediate host is a snail c. Most pigs have a natural immunity to infection
	12. Fluke (*Opisthorchis felineus*)	Intestine; bile duct; pancreatic duct	a. Low level infections: There are none b. Heavy infections: Possible inflammation and damage of the bile and pancreatic ducts	a. Don't feed raw fish to your pigs b. Give Praziquantel or Niclofan after consulting with your vet for the recommended dosage	a. This thin fluke grows to be a little under $7/10''$ long as an adult b. Its first intermediate host is a snail; the second is a fish
	13. Intestinal tapeworm of the dog (*Echinococcus granulosus*)	Intestines; liver; lungs	There are none	a. Keep dogs away from your pigs b. Don't let your pigs eat slaughterhouse wastes or any part of a pig that either dies or is slaughtered on the farm c. Check with your vet for drug treatment	a. The pig is one of several possible intermediate hosts for this tapeworm, whose final host is the dog b. Pigs become infested by eating eggs that are passed in dog feces

	Parasite	Location	Signs	Treatment/Prevention	Remarks
14.	Human tapeworm (*Taenia solium*)	Skeletal muscles; the heart	There are none	a. Good sanitary practices b. Check with your vet for drug treatment	a. The pig is an intermediate host, man is the final one that becomes infected by eating pork containing the encysted larvae b. Encysted larvae are 7/10″ long and white
15.	Kidney worm (*Stephanurus dentatus*)	Small intestine; kidney; liver; lungs; spleen; pancreas; spinal cord	a. Inflammation and damage to tissue wherever it is found b. The hindquarters may be paralyzed if the spinal cord has been injured	a. Migrating larvae may be treated by mixing Thiabendazole in the feed (454 mg/lb of feed) for 2 weeks b. Ask your vet's advice on management practices to control infection in your herd and for a recommended drug treatment	a. Adult worms are fat, black-and-white spotted, and range from 1″ to 1-2/5″ in length b. Eggs are killed by direct sunlight, extremes of temperature, and very dry weather c. Infection is through swallowing the eggs, an intermediate host, an earthworm, or by the larvae biting their way through the skin d. This parasite occurs throughout the world and is one of the most common parasites of the pig e. Sunny pastures may be considered free of kidney worms 1½ years after infected animals have been removed
16.	Coccidiosis (*Eimeria debliecki*; *E. scabra*; *E. spinosa*;	Small intestine; large intestine	a. Diarrhea b. Loss of appetite c. Loss of weight d. Poor condition	a. Proper sanitation b. Good nutrition c. Reduce stress conditions, such as over-	a. Piglets 1–3 months old are usually attacked b. Occurs off and on during rainy seasons

Animal Species	Common Name (Scientific Name)	Part of the Body Injured	Symptoms	Control and Treatment	Other Information
	Isospora suis			crowding d. Make sure pens and housing are dry and clean e. Check with your vet for recommended drug treatment	and frequently in over-crowded pens in cold weather c. Treat healthy animals preventively when individual animals show signs of infection d. It's very important to prevent dehydration e. Secondary infections may occur
	17. (*Sarcocystis suihominis; S. Porcifelis*)	Muscles; tissue lining the heart and blood vessels; nerve tissue	a. In mild infections there are no symptoms b. In serious infections: 1. Fever 2. Loss of appetite 3. Diarrhea 4. Anemia 5. Weakness 6. Wasting away 7. Collapse 8. Death	a. Don't let dogs or cats eat dead pigs or slaughter wastes b. Keep dogs and cats out of pig housing, off of their pastures, and out of feed mills and grain storage areas c. For drug treatment in case of serious in-fection check with your vet	a. Sarcocystosis is a protozoan disease b. The pig is an in-termediate host which is eaten by a final host (either a human, a dog, or cat) in order to complete the parasite's life cycle c. Pigs become infected by swallowing spores on pastures or in feed that are voided in dog, cat, or human feces

Animal Species	Common Name (Scientific Name)	Part of the Body Injured	Symptoms	Control and Treatment	Other Information
Sheep and Goats	1. Large stomach worm; Wire worm; Barber pole worm (Haemonchus contortus)	Stomach	a. Loss of weight b. Anemia c. Digestive upset d. Death	a. Rotational grazing b. Alternate grazing of different age groups c. Any of the following drugs may be used: 1. Oxfendazole given orally (2.3 mg/lb body wt) 2. Albendazole given orally (3.4 mg/lb body wt) 3. Levamisole given orally as a drench, a bolus, mixed into the feed or drinking water (2–5 mg/lb body wt) 4. Thiophanate given orally as a drench, or mixed into the feed (22–45 mg/lb body wt)	a. Found in tropical and subtropical regions and in those with summer rains b. Lactating ewes often become heavily infested, occasionally resulting in death c. Watch out for the development of drug resistance
	2. Medium stomach worm; brown stomach worm (Ostertagia circumcincta)	Stomach	a. Loss of appetite b. Digestive upsets c. Loss of weight d. Weakness e. Diarrhea and lowered milk production in ewes	a. Same drug treatment as for the large stomach worm b. Move to clean pasture	a. Found most commonly in temperate zones and where it rains in the winter b. More eggs are produced around lambing than normal. This is usually how lambs become infected c. Watch out for the development of drug resistance
	3. Small stomach	Stomach	a. Loss of appetite	a. Same drug treatment	a. Found most commonly

151

Animal Species	Common Name (Scientific Name)	Part of the Body Injured	Symptoms	Control and Treatment	Other Information
	worm (*Trichostrongylus axei*)		b. Digestive upsets c. Loss of weight d. Weakness	as for the large stomach worm b. Move to clean pasture	in the Temperate Zone and where it rains in the winter
	4. (*Trichostrongylus colubriformis; T. vitrinus; T. rugatus*)	Intestines	a. Loss of appetite b. A continuing diarrhea c. Loss of weight d. Digestive upsets	a. Same drug treatment as for the large stomach worm b. Move to clean pasture	
	5. Hookworm (*Bunostomum trigonocephalum*)	Small intestine	a. Stamping and uneasiness of animals b. Anemia c. Quick loss of weight d. Alternating diarrhea and constipation	a. Same drug treatment as above b. Move to clean pasture	a. Mature adults are about $^1/_{10}$" long b. Larvae are swallowed or can penetrate the skin
	6. Nematodes (many varieites of *Nematodirus*)	Small intestine	a. Poor condition b. Heavy diarrhea c. Dehydration d. Inflammation of small intestine e. Sudden death	a. Don't use lambing pastures 2 years in a row b. Move to clean pasture c. Same drug treatment as above	a. Eggs hatch only in wet weather. Since eggs lie dormant and continue to build up in dry conditions, large outbreaks occur 2–4 weeks after a rain b. Lambs 6–12 weeks old are most affected

	7. Nodular worm (*Oesophagostomum Columbianum*)	Intestines	a. In the early stage:
			  1. Diarrhea
			  2. Blood and mucus often seen in the feces
			  3. Weakness
			  4. Wasting away
			b. Over a period of time (several months):
			  1. Weakness
				a. Same drug treatment as above
				b. Move to clean pasture
					a. After several months, as sheep develop resistance, nodules form around larvae causing the humped back and stiff walk

		2. Loss of weight even though the animal eats well 3. Alternating diarrhea and constipation 4. Humped back and/or stiff walk		
8. Large mouth bowel worm (*Chabertia*)	Large intestine	a. Poor condition b. Soft feces filled with mucus c. Blood may be seen in the feces d. Hemorrhage of the large intestine	a. Same drug treatment as above b. Move to clean pasture	a. Immunity is acquired quickly b. Infestation occurs when animals are stressed strongly
9. Whipworm (*Trichuris*)	Large intestine	a. Poor condition b. Diarrhea c. Swelling of the large intestine	a. Don't feed on the ground during drought b. Same drug treatment as above	a. Animals rarely have bad infestations b. Infections occur in very young sheep and when animals are fed balanced feed or grain on the ground during drought
10. Tapeworm (*Moniezia expansa*)	The intestines (but only mildly, if even that)	a. In mild cases there are no symptoms b. In bad infestations animals have poorer than normal conditions and digestive upsets c. Look for yellow segments in the feces	a. Alternate age groups on pasture b. Any of the following drugs can be used for treatment: 1. Lead arsenate given orally (0.5–1 g per animal) followed by a dose of castor oil	a. The intermediate host is a mite, which is then swallowed in pasture b. This tapeworm usually only affects sheep up to 4–5 months old. After this age they're resistant

Animal Species	Common Name (Scientific Name)	Part of the Body Injured	Symptoms	Control and Treatment	Other Information
	11. Fringed tapeworm (*Thysanosoma actinioides*)	Small intestine; bile duct; pancreatic duct	and sticking out of the anus a. There are no indications of injury to the animal b. Look for pearly white, bell-shaped segments in the feces	2. Niclosamide given as a drench (35 mg/lb body wt) 3. Either Cambendazole or Albendazole orally following your vet's recommendation as to dosage a. Give niclosamide as a drench (114 mg/lb body wt)	a. This is a common tapeworm of sheep in the western part of the U.S.
	12. Sorehead; Clear-eyed blindness (*Elaeophora schneideri*)	The arteries in the head that carry blood to the brain; arteries in the spinal cord; arteries in the jaw; tiny blood vessels of the forehead and face	a. Shortly after infection: 1. Brain damage 2. Blindness 3. Incoordination, circling, and convulsions followed by rapid death b. If animals survive this first stage: 1. A bloody, raw inflammation of the forehead, face or back of the head. It's sometimes seen on the belly, legs, or hooves.	a. Control horseflies b. Give a Piperazine salt compound orally (100 mg/lb body wt). This will cure the condition in 18–20 days c. In case of brain damage there is no treatment except slaughter	a. The intermediate host is the horsefly b. The normal final hosts are several varieties of deer c. Young animals die more frequently than older ones d. Death usually takes place 3–5 weeks after larval infection and occurs very quickly

154

13. Lungworm (*Protostrongylus rufescens*; Muellerius capillaris*)	Lungs	These wounds partially heal and then erupt again for 3 years; then they heal for good a. Poor condition b. Lung tissue damage	a. Pasture different age groups separately b. Rotate pastures c. Keep animals off of swampy or marshy lands and wet areas d. Control slugs and snails by draining wet land or through specific pesticide use But be careful of risk to other animal species! e. Try spreading a mixture of 20 lbs ground copper sulfate with 80 lbs sand per acre as a preventative control f. Any of the following drugs may be used: 1. Use Cambendazole orally as a paste, a bolus, or mix it in the feed or drinking water (9–11.5 mg/lb body wt) 2. Give Fenbendazole orally (2.3 mg/lb body wt) 3. Give Oxfendazole orally (2.3 mg/lb body wt) 4. Give Albendazole	a. Larvae thrive in mild temperatures and high humidity b. Larvae can survive in the Temperate Zone for 1 year or more c. Usually affects young animals during their first year on pasture d. Intermediate hosts may be either snails or slugs

155

Animal Species	Common Name (Scientific Name)	Part of the Body Injured	Symptoms	Control and Treatment	Other Information
	14. Common liver fluke (*Fasciola hepatica*)	Intestine; liver; bile duct; lungs	a. Swollen, painful belly b. Anemia c. Soft swelling under the jaw d. Pale gums e. Wasting away f. Hemorrhage g. Rapid death	orally (3.4 mg/lb body wt) a. Keep animals off swampy, marshy and wet lands b. Control snails by draining land or with *responsible* pesticide use c. Try a preventive top dressing of 20 lbs ground copper sulfate mixed with 80 lbs of sand per acre d. Vaccinate sheep against infective necrotic hepatitis if it occurs in your area e. Regularly treat your animals each year in late fall or early winter with Rafoxanide, Brotianide, or Nitroxynil following your vet's recommendations f. If you raise cattle and sheep on the same farm treat the cattle as well	a. An acquatic snail is the intermediate host b. Heavy infestations kill both sheep and goats c. Migrating larvae that destroy liver tissue in sheep, especially 1–4 year olds, during the summer and early fall, may cause *Clostridium novyi* spores to become active. This causes a fatal blood poisoning called infectious necrotic hepatitis
	15. Giant liver fluke (*Fasciola gigantica*)	Intestine; liver; bile duct; lungs	Same as with the common liver fluke	Same as with the common liver fluke	a. Occurs in warmer areas than the common liver fluke b. Death usually occurs rapidly after infection

	Location	Symptoms	Control and prevention	Characteristics
16. Large liver fluke (*Fascioloides magna*)	Intestine; liver; bile duct; other organs	a. Destruction of liver tissue b. Rapid death	a. Control and prevention are the same as with the common liver fluke b. Keep deer fenced out of sheep grazing lands c. Check with your vet for drug treatment	a. Deer are the usual hosts and are necessary for egg production b. Larvae migrate widely, causing enormous tissue damage

17. Lancet fluke; lesser liver fluke (*Dicrocoelium dendriticum*)	Intestine; liver; bile duct	a. In mild infection no symptoms are seen
		b. In heavy infestations:
		  1. Jaundice may occur
		  2. The bile duct thickens and swells
		  3. Liver damage occurs
			a. Control and preventative measures are the same as with the common liver fluke
			b. Use Hetolin, Thiabendazole or Praziquantel following your vet's recommendation
				a. Adult flukes are ½″ long and thin
				b. The first intermediate host is a snail; the second is an ant

18. Pancreatic fluke (*Eurytrema pancreaticum; E. coelomaticum; E. ovis*)	Pancreatic duct and sometimes the bile duct	a. The pancreatic duct is swollen and may be badly damaged	a. Control and prevention are the same as with the common liver fluke b. Use Praziquantel, a benzimidazole or follow your vet's recommendation	a. The adult is ⅗″ long and ¼″ wide b. This fluke is widely distributed in Asia and Brazil c. The first intermediate host is a snail; the second is a grasshopper
19. Stomach fluke (There are many species)	Small intestine; rumen; recticulum	Fluke larvae cause: a. Bad inflammation of the small intestine b. Loss of appetite c. Tremendous thirst d. Bad diarrhea e. Death (especially in young animals)	a. Control and prevention are the same as with the common liver fluke b. Use Resorantel according to the manufacturer's instructions	a. Adults are ⅗″ long, pink or red and look like tiny pears b. The intermediate host is a snail

Animal Species	Common Name (Scientific Name)	Part of the Body Injured	Symptoms	Control and Treatment	Other Information
20.	Blood fluke (Caused by many species of *Schistosomes*)	The intestines; liver; blood vessels; bladder; pancreas	a. Blood flukes of the intestine and liver: 1. Anemia 2. Inflammation and hemorrhage of the intestines 3. Wasting away 4. Death	a. Control and prevention are the same as with the common liver fluke b. Use Trichlorfon, hydrochloride, hycanthone, lucanthone, or Stibophen under the direction of your vet	a. Adults are very thin, 1½" long, and found in blood cells b. This fluke is found in several countries along the Mediterranean Sea, in Africa, Asia, the Middle East, and the Caribbean c. The intermediate host is an acuatic snail
21.	Tapeworm (*Taenia multiceps*)	Brain	a. Inflammation of the brain b. Excessive sleepiness c. Loss of appetite d. Wasting away e. Circling or turning movements f. Stumbling walk	a. Keep dogs fenced out of sheep pastures b. Consult with your vet	a. The definitive hosts are the dog, fox, and jackel b. *Taenia* causes a disease commonly called gid or staggers, named for the uncoordinated effect it causes in sheep due to brain damage c. Sheep become infected by consuming *taenia* segments, in pasture, that have been passed in dog feces
22.	Intestinal tapeworm of the dog (*Echinococcus granulosus*)	Liver; lungs; other tissues and organs	There are none	a. Keep dogs, foxes, and wolves fenced out of sheep pastures b. Don't let dogs eat dead sheep on the range or any part of a sheep slaughtered on the farm	a. The definitive host is the dog, which becomes infected by eating infested sheep guts, usually on the range b. Sheep are infected by

23. Coccidiosis (*Eimeria ahsata*; *E. ninakohlyaki-movae*; *E. cran-dallis*; *E. faurei*; *E. arloingli*; *E. parua*)	Small intestine; large intestine	a. Mild infections:
		  1. Reduced appetite
		  2. Mild diarrhea
		b. Serious infections:
		  1. Bad diarrhea
		  2. Straining to pass feces
		  3. Feces are bloody and dark colored
		  4. Loss of appetite
		  5. Loss of weight
		  6. 10% of animals die
			a. Proper sanitation
			b. Good nutrition and fresh, clean water
			c. Reduce stress conditions, such as feed lot overcrowding
			d. For preventative treatment of lambs in feedlots:
			  1. Mix 1 gm of sulfaguanidine with each pound of grain or chopped hay fed during the first month of feedlot confinement
			  2. Mix sodium arsanilate or arsanilic acid into the feed (45 mg/lb of feed) for the first month in the feedlot
			e. Any of the following drugs can be used for treatment:
			  1. Give sulfaquinox-aline orally for 3–5 days (6 mg/lb body wt)
			  2. Give sulfamerazine solution orally (60
				a. Of pasture animals, lambs 1–3 months old are the worst affected
				b. Worst infections occur to feedlot lambs 2–4 weeks after entering the lot
				c. When infection occurs in a feedlot treat healthy animals preventatively
				d. It's important to prevent dehydration
				e. Secondary infections, like pneumonia, occur often

Additional notes (from adjacent row, top):
swallowing tapeworm segments on pasture that were voided in dog feces

c. Check with your vet for drug treatment

Animal Species	Common Name (Scientific Name)	Part of the Body Injured	Symptoms	Control and Treatment	Other Information
				mg/lb body wt). Follow this dose with 30 mg/lb body wt every 24 hrs for 4 days 3. Sulfamethazine orally or IV (100 mg/lb body wt on the first day. Starting the second day give 50 mg/lb of body wt for 3–4 days)	
	24. (*Sarcocystis ovicanis; S. Tenella*)	Muscles; tissue lining the heart and blood vessels; nerve tissue	a. In mild infections there are no symptoms b. In serious infections: 1. Fever 2. Loss of appetite 3. Diarrhea 4. Anemia 5. Weakness 6. Wasting away 7. Abortion 8. Collapse 9. Death	a. Don't let dogs or cats eat dead sheep or slaughter wastes b. Keep dogs and cats off of sheep pasture and out of feedlots, feed mills, and grain storage areas c. In case of serious infection check with your vet for drug treatment	a. Sarcocystosis is a protozoan disease b. Sheep are intermediate hosts which are eaten by final hosts (dog or cat) in order to complete the parasite's life cycle c. Sheep become infected by swallowing spores on pasture or in feed that are voided in dog or cat feces
Rabbits	1. Coccidiosis of the liver (*Eimeria stiedai*)	Liver	a. Diarrhea b. Loss of appetite c. The fur becomes rough d. Poor growth e. Weakness	a. Good sanitation b. Cages must be dry and clean of feces c. Prevent stress conditions d. For preventative treatment use sulfaquinoxaline:	a. Young rabbits are most seriously affected b. Rabbits cured of this protozoan disease usually remain carriers c. When using sulfaquinoxaline for prevention or treatment

160

Disease	Location	Symptoms	Treatment	Remarks
			1. Mix into the feed (113.5 mg/lb of feed) for 20 days, or 2. Mix into the drinking water (at a concentration of 0.025%) for 30 days e. For treatment in case of infection use sulfaquinoxaline: 1. Mixed into the feed (454 mg/lb of feed) for 2 weeks or 2. Mixed both into the feed (227 mg/lb of feed) and into the drinking water (at a concentration of 0.04%) for 2 weeks	discontinue use for at least 10 days before slaughter
2. Coccidiosis of the intestine (Eimeria magna; E. irresidua; E. media; E. perforans)	Intestines	a. Loss of appetite b. Poor growth c. Swollen belly d. Diarrhea e. Weakness	a. Good sanitation b. Prevent stress conditions c. Treat infected animals with sulfaquinoxaline mixed into the feed (454 mg/lb of feed) for 2 weeks	a. Intestinal coccidiosis must be treated for separately from coccidiosis of the liver
3. Dog tapeworm (Taenia pisiformis)	Intestines; internal organs	a. Poor growth b. Diarrhea c. Blood or mucus in the feces	a. Good sanitation b. Don't let dogs eat rabbit slaughter wastes c. Keep dogs away from rabbit hutches, feed, and drinking water d. Check with your vet for drug treatment	a. The rabbit is an intermediate host for the larval stage b. Rabbits become infected by eating eggs passed in dog feces that get into food and water or onto pans, feeders, hutches, and so forth

Animal Species	Common Name (Scientific Name)	Part of the Body Injured	Symptoms	Control and Treatment	Other Information
	4. Dog tapeworm (*Taenia serialis*)	Intestines; internal organs	Same as above	Same as above	Same as above
	5. Cat tapeworm (*Taenia Taeniaeformis*)	Liver	Same as above	a. Good sanitation b. Don't let cats eat rabbit slaughter wastes c. Keep cats away from rabbit hutches, feed, and drinking water d. Check with your vet for a drug treatment	a. The rabbit is an intermediate host for the larval stage b. Rabbits become infected by eating eggs passed in cat feces that get into food and water or onto pans, feeders, hutches, and so on
	6. Nosematosis (*Nosemacuniculi*)	Brain; kidney	No symptoms are seen	a. Good sanitation b. Check with your vet for drug treatment	a. Nosematosis is a common contagious protozoan disease of rabbits
	7. Pinworm (*Passalurus ambiguus*)	Large intestine; rectum	a. Rubbing of the tail and anus	a. Good sanitation b. Mix phenothiazine into feed made with molasses (1 g/50 g of feed)	
Poultry	1. Coccidiosis (Chicken, 9 varieties: turkey, 7 varieties; duck, at least 7 varieties; goose, at least 6 varieties)	Intestines; 1 variety in the goose attacks the kidneys	Symptoms vary according to variety, but the following is a general guide: a. Chickens: 1. Blood in the feces 2. Dehydration 3. Crop swollen with water 4. Poor growth 5. Bad diarrhea 6. Loss of weight 7. Reduced egg	a. Good sanitary conditions b. Clean, dry housing c. Keep birds on wire floors to prevent contamination with their feces d. Treat preventively by maintaining low drug level in drinking water e. Keep birds separated	a. Most common disease of poultry b. Purposefully allowing mild infection helps develop immunity to this protozoan c. Younger birds more seriously affected than older ones d. Look for signs of drug resistance and if seen

change treatment

by age group

f. Sulfanamide drugs are best for treatment. Check with your vet for recommended drug and dosage for each poultry species

     laying
8. Pale comb and wattles
9. Don't move around as much as normal
10. Death

b. Turkeys:
1. Droopy looking
2. Ruffled feathers
3. Lowered feed consumption
4. Serious loss of weight
5. Bad diarrhea
6. Wetter than normal feces containing mucus
7. Death

c. Ducks:
1. Inflammation and hemorrhage of the intestines
2. Loss of weight
3. Diarrhea
4. Reduced feed consumption
5. Death

d. Geese:
1. Loss of weight
2. Reduced feed consumption
3. Diarrhea
4. Death

Animal Species	Common Name (Scientific Name)	Part of the Body Injured	Symptoms	Control and Treatment	Other Information
	2. Gapeworm (Syngamus trachea in chickens and turkeys; Cyathostoma bronchialis in ducks and geese)	Windpipe; lungs	a. Grasping and choking b. Sneezing c. Shaking the head d. Coughing e. Loss of appetite f. Wasting away g. Suffocation h. Pneumonia i. Rapid death	a. Keep birds off freshly plowed fields b. Don't let birds out into pens or runs until the dew is gone and no earthworms are seen c. Good sanitation d. Control slugs, snails, and earthworms e. Keep birds off wetlands f. Preventative treatment: 　1. Thiabendazole mixed into the feed (227 mg/lb of feed) for 4 days or longer g. Treatment in case of infection: 　1. Thiabendazole mixed into the feed (454 mg/lb of feed) for 10–14 days 　2. Tetramisole mixed into the drinking water (1.6 mg/lb body wt) for 3 days	a. Infection is via eggs and larvae in the soil, feed and litter, as well as many intermediate hosts (snails, slugs, earthworms, flies) b. Young birds are most severely affected c. Immunity is developed after surviving an attack
	3. Blackhead; Histomoniasis (Histomonas Meleagridis)	Liver; intestines	a. Turkeys: 　1. Droopy looking 　2. No energy 　3. Ruffled feathers 　4. Loss of appetite 　5. Greater than normal thirst 　6. Yellow colored feces	a. Good sanitation b. Keep chickens and turkeys separated, both in housing and in pens c. Don't let turkeys range on land chickens have been on and vice versa d. Keep young birds separated from older	a. Blackhead is a protozoan disease of turkeys and chickens b. Infection takes place by swallowing eggs passed in the feces or by swallowing eggs of the cecal worm which contain histomonas

eggs

c. Symptoms appear 1–2 weeks after infection
d. Young birds are most severely affected but older ones become infected as well
e. 80–90% of young turkeys 1–3 months old die when infected

ones

e. Keep birds off of contaminated range for 1–2 years
f. Range-fed turkeys should be rotated to fresh ground every 3–5 weeks
g. Mix Phenothiazine or tobacco dust into the feed to get rid of cecal worms. Follow manufacturer's recommendations. (This won't kill the histomas protozoa.)
h. Preventive treatment in turkeys:
   1. Mix Ronidazole into the feed (27–54 mg/lb of feed) or
   2. Mix Furazolidone into the feed (50 mg/lb of feed) or
   3. Mix carbarsone into the feed (170 mg/lb of feed). Stop feeding this drug 5 days before birds go to market, or
   4. Mix Dimetridazole into the feed (225 mg/lb of feed). Stop feeding this drug 5 days before birds go to market
i. For treatment in case of infection in turkeys use any of the following drugs:

7. The head may turn dark in color
8. Loss of weight
9. Death
b. Chickens rarely show obvious symptoms

Animal Species	Common Name (Scientific Name)	Part of the Body Injured	Symptoms	Control and Treatment	Other Information
				1. Mix Dimetridazole powder into the drinking water (1.25 g/liter of water) for 6 days. Then continue with preventative treatment (h4)—see above 2. Mix Nitrasone into the feed (82 mg/lb of feed). Stop feeding this drug 5 days before birds go to market 3. Mix Furazolidone into the feed (75 mg/lb of feed) for 2–3 weeks	

4.	Manson's eyeworm (*Oxyspirura mansoni*)	Eye; nasal passage	a. Inflammation of the eye
			b. Tears in the eyes
			c. The outer membrane of the eye changes from transparent to opaque
			d. Difficulty seeing
				a. Good sanitation
				b. Control of cockroaches through use of insecticide
				c. Preventative treatment (done by your vet):
				  1. Surgically removing the inner eyelid
				d. Treatment in case of infection (done by your vet):
				  1. After anesthetizing the eye, lift the inner eyelid and put 1–2 drops of creosol solution (5% concentration) in the
					a. Manson's eyeworm is a thin roundworm 1/2"–7/10" long found under the inner eyelid in chickens
					b. It occurs in semi-tropical and tropical zones
					c. The intermediate host is a cockroach

No. / Disease	Location	Symptoms	Treatment	Remarks
			tear ducts. This kills the worms Wash the eye out right away with clean water. Eyesight will improve 2–3 days after this and the eye's outer membrane will slowly become transparent again if not too much permanent damage has been done.	

5. Hexamitiasis (*Hexamitamelea-gridis*)	Small intestine	a. Watery, foamy diarrhea
		b. Droopy looking
		c. No energy
		d. Dry ruffled feathers
		e. Sudden loss of weight though animals may still eat
		f. Stiff walk
		g. Lower than normal body temperature
		h. Death (sometimes with convulsions)
			a. Good sanitation
			b. Young and adult turkeys should be raised in separate housing by different workers. They should have separate ranges
			c. Preventive treatment:
			  1. Mix Furazolidone into the feed (25 mg/lb of feed)
			d. For treatment in case of infection any of the following drugs may be used:
			  1. Mix chlortetracycline into the feed (100–200 mg/lb of feed) for 2 weeks
			  2. Mix oxytetracycline into the feed (100 mg/lb of feed) for 2 weeks
				a. Hexamitiasis is a protozoan disease in turkeys acquired by eating feces that contain infective spores
				b. It was once widespread in North America but is now rare
				c. Birds 1 week to 3 months old are the most severely affected
				d. Surviving birds may be carriers

Animal Species	Common Name (Scientific Name)	Part of the Body Injured	Symptoms	Control and Treatment	Other Information
	6. Leucocytozoon disease (Chickens: *Leucocytozoon sabrazesi*; *L. caulleryi*; *L. andrewsi*; Turkeys: *L. smithi*; ducks and geese: *L. simondi*)	Blood vessels; body tissues	a. In general: 1. Loss of appetite 2. Birds are sleepy looking, but if forced to move they become overexcited, may lose their balance and go into convulsions 3. Weakness 4. Loss of balance 5. Anemia 6. Death b. In chickens severely attacked by *L. caulleryi*: 1. Anemia 2. May vomit 3. Sometimes green feces are seen 4. Possible death from hemorrhage, anemia, liver, brain or respiratory damage 5. Surviving chickens show poor growth and lower than normal egg production	3. Fix furazolidone into the feed (50 mg/lb of feed) for 2–3 weeks a. Locate poultry farms away from swampy, wet areas and fast moving streams where midges and black flies breed b. If feasible, tightly screen housing c. In affected zones raise turkeys and ducks inside. Black flies generally only feed outside d. Raise turkeys to maturity and sell them off before fly season e. Any of the following drugs may be used for preventive treatment with chickens exposed to *L. caulleryi*: 1. Mix pyrimethamine into the feed (227 mg/1,000 lbs of feed) 2. Mix sulfadimethoxine into the feed (11.35 mg/lb of feed) or the drinking water (at a 0.0025% concentration) 3. Mix sulfaquinoxaline into the feed (22.7 mg/lb of feed) or the	a. The disease is caused by protozoa (similar to those that cause malaria) and spread by black flies and biting midges (in one of the species that attacks chickens) b. Heavy infection occurs during fly season in late spring and summer c. Young turkeys up to 3 months old and ducklings 2–8 weeks old are most heavily attacked

	Location	Symptoms	Prevention/Control	Description
			drinking water (at a 0.005% concentration) f. There is no known drug treatment for other leucocytozoon species	
7. Fluke (*Prosthogonimum macrorchis*)	Oviduct (one of a pair of tubes through which eggs pass from the ovary)	a. Serious infections in the chicken and turkey: 1. Droopyness 2. Reduced appetite 3. Loss of weight 4. Egg laying is reduced or stops altogether 5. Eggs have soft shells 6. A chalky fluid covers the feathers around the *cloaca* (anus) 7. Possible rupture of the oviduct 8. Death	a. Keep birds away from lakes, ponds, streams, marshes, and swamps and any wet area, where dragonflies are found b. There is presently no recommended drug treatment but check with your vet to see if something new has come out on the market	a. This fluke is pear-shaped and about ¼″ long b. The first host is a snail; the second is an immature dragonfly, which birds eat and become infected by.
8. (*Collyriclum faba*)	Under the surface of the skin	a. Reduced appetite b. Uncoordinated movements c. Oozing fluid from the cysts under the skin d. Death, in bad infections	a. Keep birds out of wet areas where dragonflies or mayflies are found b. There is presently no recommended drug treatment but check with your vet	a. The intermediate hosts are suspected to be a snail and a dragonfly or mayfly b. The parasite lives in a cyst under the surface of the skin, especially near the anus

16

GENERAL DISEASES OF DOMESTIC ANIMALS

Anthrax

Anthrax is an infectious and often fatal disease that attacks warm-blooded animals throughout the world. It is caused by a very powerful and fast-acting bacteria. Of the domestic farm animals, cattle, horses, mules, sheep, goats, pigs, and rabbits are the most severely affected. Once bacteria enter an animal's body they grow very quickly, multiply, and penetrate the bloodstream. *Septicemia*, a blood infection, usually results and the animal dies within a few days.

The bacteria create spores, highly resistant reproductive forms of the microorganism, when they pass from an infected animal's body in its normal discharges or when an animal that has died of anthrax is opened for an autopsy or by a scavenger as it feeds upon the carcass. Anthrax spores need oxygen, moisture, and a warm temperature to develop; once formed they are able to survive for many years despite extreme heat, cold, or dry weather, and are resistant to powerful chemical disinfectants. Spores in infected regions are commonly found in the soil, on pastures, and in the drinking water, but may be carried great distances from the areas where the disease has occurred by the wind, insects, and scavengers. Spores are also found in animal products, such as hides and bristles, from infected animals, and in feeds and feed ingredients such as bonemeal and meat scraps produced from animals that have died of anthrax.

Human beings become infected by coming in contact with the blood or tissues of diseased animals, by inhaling spores while working with hides and other infected animal by-products, or by eating diseased meat.

Infection

Domestic farm animals usually become infected while grazing on anthrax-contaminated pastures or when consuming contaminated feed. Infections often occur on diseased pastures as grass becomes less plentiful and is grazed closer to the ground in late summer and early fall. Such pastures are generally found on neutral-alkaline, chalky soils. Outbreaks invariably occur during warm weather and especially when the weather changes dramatically. Anthrax infections can be expected in disease-prone areas when an extended drought is ended with a strong downpour.

Cattle, horses, mules, sheep, goats, and rabbits are very susceptible to infection; pigs and humans have a stronger resistance to the disease and are less often infected.

Symptoms

Anthrax symptoms depend upon the type of animal and the rapidity with which it is infected. Anthrax can also appear as a chronic or local infection in some types of animals.

Very Rapid (Peracute) Infection

This is most common in cattle, sheep, and goats that haven't shown any prior signs of disease. In this form the disease closely resembles a brain hemorrhage: all of a sudden animals have difficulty breathing, they stagger, tremble uncontrollably, fall down, move convulsively a few times, and die. The whole sequence of symptoms occurs very quickly, sometimes taking no more than a matter of minutes.

Rapid (Acute) Infection

Cattle, horses, and sheep body temperatures rise (eventually they may reach 107°F. [41.5°C]) and they become excited and agitated. After this they become depressed, sink into a stupor, and have difficulty breathing. Their heart beats irregularly and they stagger, collapse, go into convulsions, and then die. During the day or two it takes animals to die, milk production drops drastically. Different parts of the body swell up, animals may bleed from the nostrils, mouth, vagina, penis, or anus and females may abort.

In addition to these symptoms horses may develop a fever or chills, have strong abdominal pains, lose their appetites, and become very depressed. A bloody diarrhea is sometimes seen, and the neck, the region around the breastbone, the lower belly, vulva, penis, and testicles may become swollen. In general, muscles lose their tone and become weak.

Hogs occasionally die of the acute form of anthrax without showing any symptoms of infection. In other cases loss of appetite, vomiting, and bloody diarrhea are seen. Animals also swell up quickly around the throat and may suffocate, gasping for breath.

Long-Lasting (Chronic) Infection

Chronic infections occur most often in hogs, but can also affect horses and cattle, although only infrequently. Wounds of the tongue and throat are seen; recovery takes a long time.

Local Infection

When anthrax bacteria invade wounds and skin injuries in cattle and horses those parts of their bodies become swollen. This is not a fatal form of the disease when treated promptly and if not allowed to develop into septicemia. It is often caused by the bites of infected flies or when animals that are susceptible to the disease are vaccinated.

Treatment of the Carcass

After death from anthrax dark blood often seeps from the nostrils and anus. The body bloats and quickly rots. Rigor mortis, the stiffening of the body after death, either doesn't happen at all or only partially. *Never attempt to do an autopsy or to remove blood or tissue samples from an animal suspected of having died of anthrax.*

If death from anthrax is suspected, you should call your veterinarian and ask him or her to take the necessary samples; they are trained to do this and know how to take the proper precautions so as to not become infected by the microorganisms present in the blood or tissues.

Diagnoses Should Be Based on Laboratory Examination

The diagnosis of anthrax from the disease symptoms shown by an animal is never considered to be reliable without confirmation from a laboratory analysis. In each stage of infection anthrax symptoms are similar to those produced by other diseases or natural causes of sudden death.

In cattle symptoms may be confused with those of anaplasmosis (an infectious, often fatal disease of the blood), being hit by lightning, bloat, lead poisoning, sweet clover and bracken fern poisonings, clostridium infections (caused by powerful bacteria that need an absence of air to thrive and multiply), severe leptospirosis (a bacterial disease in which blood cells are destroyed and fetuses abort), and brain hemorrhage.

In horses symptoms are sometimes mistaken for those of lead poisoning, sunstroke, severe infectious anemia, several kinds of colics (severe abdominal pains), and being hit by lightning. The signs of bloat, being hit by lighting, and clostridium infections are similar to those of anthrax in sheep. In pigs symptoms are like those of severe hog cholera and malignant edema (a serious and usually fatal blood poisoning characterized by the swelling of different parts of the body).

Control Measures

Anthrax control is effected by an annual preventive vaccination with an antianthrax vaccine and by close attention to the following measures in the case of disease outbreak:

1. Inform the proper health authorities if anthrax is either suspected or confirmed.
2. Quarantine infected herds and farms.

3. The carcasses of animals that die on pasture, range, or away from buildings should be completely burned without moving them.
4. If for some reason it's not possible to burn the carcass, dig a pit at least 4 feet deep. Roll the carcass into it, cover it liberally with lime, and fill in the pit with dirt.
5. Burn all materials contaminated by an animal with anthrax; this includes manure, litter, bedding, and poles used to roll a carcass into a pit for deep burial.
6. Disinfect all housing, pens, stables, enclosures, floors, and tools that diseased animals have come in contact with. To do this prepare a fresh solution of hot lye (5 percent sodium hydroxide mixed with water). Observe all warnings and manufacturer's instructions for preparation and use.
7. Isolate all diseased animals and treat them with antibiotics.
8. Vaccinate all apparently healthy animals in a herd that has been infected with anthrax and those herds in the surrounding area.
9. Move apparently healthy animals to an uncontaminated area and observe them for disease symptoms. Keep them isolated from other herds.
10. Use insect repellents to prevent anthrax transmission by biting insects.
11. Never allow an animal that is suspected to have died of anthrax to be opened for autopsy or to have tissue or blood samples taken by anyone who is not a veterinarian. Never skin these animals.
12. Prevent scavengers from feeding on animals that have died or are suspected to have died of anthrax.
13. Anyone who must handle the carcass of an animal that has died from anthrax should wear rubber gloves, rubber boots, and a long rain jacket. Afterward these should all be properly disinfected.

Treatment

Treatment in the early stage of infection can save and cure animals depending on the severity of outbreak. Penicillin and oxytetracycline give the best results; dosage varies according to the animal species, the severity of disease, and the level of natural resistance. Always consult with your veterinarian for the proper treatment of your infected animals.

Foot-and-Mouth Disease

Foot-and-mouth disease, (FMD), also called aphthous fever, and *aftosa*, is a severe and very infectious viral disease of cloven-hooved animals throughout the world. FMD is a major problem in many countries in sheep, goats, cattle, and pigs, and exists in several different forms. Roughly speaking, 6 out of every 100 infected animals die of the disease, yet every once in a while half of an infected herd will suddenly be wiped out through the destruction of their heart muscles. Young animals die in greater numbers than adults, but all ages are equally susceptible to infection.

Animals become infected in a variety of ways, chief among them being direct physical contact with other diseased animals. Other mechanical means by which FMD spreads are also important: the virus may be carried from farm to farm by vehicles, tools, and workers, wild animals (especially rats and birds), flies, and other insects. The FMD virus is exhaled by animals in their breath and may be carried long distances by the wind. It survives in this microscopic water vapor mist, in the absence of sunlight and high temperatures, for a few hours, which is usually long enough to infect a susceptible herd downwind from a farm with an outbreak.

Since FMD virus is excreted into milk, saliva, urine, and feces, and is found in the animal's blood, bone, meat, skin, and hair, either physical contact with or consumption of any of these products will facilitate the spread of and infection by the disease. The use of semen from infected bulls for artificial insemination is thought to be another way the disease is transmitted. This is a particularly hard source of infection to control since cows may have been bred before the bull showed any signs of disease.

The severity of infection is dependent on the strain of the virus, the susceptibility to disease of your animals, and the proper environmental factors (these include darkness, cool temperatures, and a neutral pH). Viruses are quickly rendered noninfective by bright sunshine, high temperatures, either high or low pH, and some chemical pollutants.

Symptoms

After an animal is infected the virus incubates and develops within its body for 2-5 days before any symptoms are seen. In rapidly occurring (acute) infection the first sign of disease is a high fever; this is rarely seen in less severe outbreaks. Small white-colored blisters appear in the mouth and continue growing until they are large and swollen. The blisters are filled with either clear or pale yellow liquid, and cover the tongue, the inside of the lips and cheeks, the roof and the floor of the mouth, and the gums. The animal responds by secreting an excessive amount of saliva and looks as if it is drooling heavily. As it opens and closes its mouth it may make a smacking or slobbering sound. Because it hurts to chew, feed consumption is reduced or stops entirely. Animals lose weight and show poor, unthrifty body conditions.

Blisters also erupt on one or both feet, usually in between or just above the hoofs. Feet become hot, swollen, and very painful. Generally, animals become lame or lose their hooves. Blisters may also be seen on the udder, teats, vulva, muzzle or snout, and nostrils. These swollen, fluid-filled sacs burst within a day or two, leaving a raw wound that heals quickly. Secondary bacterial invaders may attack these raw spots, especially when they occur on the feet or udder. These secondary invaders occasionally cause mastitis, abortion, blood poisoning, or pneumonia. The normal milk production of lactating females drops noticeably or ceases altogether.

A Caution about Identification

A positive diagnosis of FMD is only possible after a laboratory examination of a virus sample removed from an infected animal. The collection of the sample should be done by your veterinarian or an authorized representative of your county's foot-and-mouth disease control and eradication program.

The symptoms of FMD are similar to those of vesicular stomatitis (a viral disease causing blisters in pigs' feet, snouts, and mouths that has only been identified in the United States and that was eradicated in 1959), and swine vesicular disease (an infection causing blisters of the feet and mouth in pigs in Western Europe, Hong Kong, and Japan).

Prevention

In those countries considered free of foot-and-mouth disease, such as the United States (the last outbreak occurred in 1929) and Canada (the last outbreak took place in 1952), prevention is dependent on very strict controls on the importation of animals and animal products from countries where the disease still exists. Only rarely are live animals allowed to be imported, and then only after a thorough laboratory examination and a strict quarantine period are observed.

Animal products such as meat, meat scraps, hides, dried blood, dried milk, bonemeal, natural casings, glands, all milk products, and animal feeds must be certified to have been safely processed in accordance with the laws of the FMD-free country or are processed at their destination under the supervision of the proper regulatory agency. Garbage containing meat or milk products that arrives from an FMD-infected country aboard any means of transport is often not allowed into the disease-free country or is immediately disposed of in an approved way. Luggage arriving from FMD-infected countries is examined at the port of entry in a disease-free country and may be confiscated and destroyed if found to be infected.

All this may sound quite drastic and it is meant to, since the effects of this disease are economically disastrous. Before the last outbreak in England was brought under control in 1968 more than 430,000 animals had to be slaughtered. The best prevention of foot-and-mouth disease is to not let it be introduced into a disease-free region.

Control Measures

The following is a list of control measures that are used in FMD-free countries and those, such as Britain, that have decided it is economically feasible to attempt to achieve that goal.

1. Quick identification of the specific strain of FMD through laboratory examination.
2. Report the disease outbreak to the local, state, and federal authorities responsible for the control and eradication of FMD.
3. Upon positive confirmation of the disease a strict quarantine of the infected farm must be established. No person or vehicle from that farm should be allowed to leave the premises until 2 weeks after the disease has been eradicated. Surrounding farms should be inspected and quarantined if necessary.
4. Infected and susceptible animals that have come in contact with those that have the disease should be slaughtered and their carcasses burned.

5. A 2 percent lye solution (sodium hydroxide) or another disinfectant recommended by your veterinarian is used to disinfect all housing, enclosures, fencing, floors, machinery, tools, clothing, and other items that may have come in contact with the virus.
6. All straw, bedding, litter, and manure must be burned.
7. After waiting a month and a half after the slaughter, clean-up, and disinfection restock the farm with a few "test" animals that are susceptible to infection with FMD. These "test" animals should come in contact with all fields, housing, enclosures, tools, machinery, and other objects that could have been contaminated with the virus. If any of these animals come down with the disease you know the cleaning and disinfection were not thorough enough and will have to be repeated.

In countries where the disease is common and control by slaughter is not possible due to economic constraints, a preventive vaccination of your animals should be carried out. Vaccinations generally last 4–6 months and must be repeated to maintain protection. Entire regions should be vaccinated en masse to develop larger and larger disease-free areas. All infected farms should be quarantined and neighboring farms considered suspect. The animals of neighboring farms must be assumed to be susceptible to infection and are closely observed for any symptoms of the disease.

Treatment of FMD only gets rid of its symptoms, it doesn't cure the animal or prevent the spread of infection. Those animals that recover from FMD are immune to reinfection for 6 months to 2 years. They may be carriers of the virus during that time, but so far there is no evidence to show that they infect other susceptible animals they come in contact with.

Brucellosis

Brucellosis is an infectious bacterial disease in cattle, hogs, sheep, goats, horses, and humans distributed throughout the world. It is one of the leading causes of abortion and reproductive failure of both sexes. There are several different types of the bacteria, yet each animal species is attacked by one principal variety, except horses which are infected by two. Man is infected by the same brucella organism as goats are; the human disease is commonly known as *undulant fever* or *malta fever*.

Infection usually occurs from eating feed or drinking water that has been contaminated with bacteria-laden discharges (milk, saliva, and urine) of animals suffering from brucellosis. Herdmates often lick each other's genitals, passing the disease among themselves. When breeding stock are held together and one or more aborts, the fetus, fetal discharge, and membranes are licked or eaten, infecting all stock that come in contact with them. Infected, lactating mothers pass the disease along to their suckling young in their milk. Boars, rams, stallions, billy goats, and occasionally bulls may infect females with bacteria carried in their semen during natural service.

The bacteria may survive for a few weeks out of the body (in manure, on litter, or wherever farm animals are found) as long as the temperature is cool and they are out of the direct sun. Hence, an animal's contact with its normal, but contaminated environment may cause infection, especially as the brucellae microorganisms are capable of penetrating both injured and healthy skin, nasal mucous membranes (when urine or milk mists are breathed in), and those of the eyes.

Infection and Symptoms

Cattle

The symptoms of brucellosis in cattle, also called contagious abortion and Bang's disease, depend on whether the herd has ever been infected by *Brucella abortus* or vaccinated before. In an unvaccinated, never infected herd, brucellae bacteria spread very quickly and cause a large number of abortions. In unvaccinated herds with continual high levels of infection, diseased animals usually abort only once but may remain infective carriers their whole lives. Animals infect their herdmates with bacterial discharges passed in their milk and urine and may have trouble being bred back following abortion. Usually, subsequent pregnancies and births are normal, although bacteria are passed from the uterus when the young are born. Bacteria are passed in the milk for long periods of time after infection.

The existence of and degree of infection depend, of course, on whether an animal has been vaccinated or not, but also to a large extent on natural resistance. Some cows have a naturally strong resistance to infection whereas others abort over and over again or are "problem breeders" that have difficulty settling (becoming pregnant when bred).

Before sexual maturity cattle are usually resistant to infection. This resistance becomes weaker and weaker as they mature and are bred. Pregnant, unvaccinated cattle are very prone to brucellosis, much more so than nonpregnant animals. Once an animal with poor resistance has been infected the bacteria pass into the bloodstream and are transported to specific organs and tissues where they further develop and increase in number. In cows the uterus, udder, spleen, and lymph glands (tissue containing white blood cells that provide immunity to infection and that fight bacterial invasion) are brucellae multiplication sites. In bulls the spleen, lymph glands, and testicles are affected.

Pregnant females abort or have weak, sickly calves; they often retain their placentas, which leads to secondary bacterial invasions. A vaginal discharge is seen and animals are generally infertile for a short time, though this may become permanent. Milk production drops by 20–25 percent due to disrupted milking cycles from abortion and breeding problems.

If cattle are artificially inseminated with brucellosis-infected semen that is deposited into the uterus, they too become infected and fail to become pregnant time after time. These "repeat breeders" may end up infecting a clean dairy bull which is used to breed them as a last hope before they are culled from the herd. Take care not to let this happen. Nonpregnant mature cows that are infected usually don't show any signs of disease.

Since brucellae multiply in bulls' reproductive organs it seems logical that they should pass into the semen. Bulls may not show outward signs of infection, but if they do you will notice that one or both of their testicles is larger than normal (a condition called *orchitis*), that they lose their sexual drive, and that their breedings don't cause pregnancy. Dairy bulls are not as prone to brucellosis attack as cows are because usually they are separated from the rest of the herd for obvious management reasons. They don't often come in contact with brucellae bacteria, except when being used to breed infected cows.

Pigs

Pigs are also infected, like cattle, by eating feed or drinking water contaminated with discharges containing brucellae. When an infected pregnant sow in a group of breeding stock aborts, the fetus, fetal fluid, and membranes are licked or eaten by the other animals. This is certain to happen since pigs are very curious animals, and it will result in the infection of the whole lot. Sows and gilts (young sows that haven't had their first litter yet) may be infected by diseased boars via their semen in natural service or when inseminated artificially. Since bacteria are shed in the sow's milk, she infects a few of her suckling piglets, but most make it to weaning without having become diseased. *Brucella suis* bacteria, the main type that attacks pigs, also enters the animal through the membranes of its eyes, the mucous membranes of its nasal passage, and through wounds and unbroken, healthy skin.

After infection brucellae follow the same course of development within the pig's body as they do in cattle. The bacteria concentrate in the lymph glands, spleen, liver, and testicles.

Abortion is the most common sign of disease and may or may not be seen depending on the stage of the pregnancy at which the infection occurs. Usually, several females bred at the same time that come into heat again (that show signs of estrus—sexual receptivity) 1 to 1-½ months after service are the first clue that your herd has brucellosis. When the abortion occurs as early as this there is practically no vaginal discharge. Later abortions are characterized by visible discharges which contain bacteria.

Animals may become either temporarily or permanently infertile. These are the "repeat breeders" that so often are culled when the farmer gives up on them in disgust after they don't settle a couple of times in a row. Infected boars lose sexual drive and one of their testicles may be larger than normal. They may become infertile and normally don't recover from a genital brucellosis infection because of the damage done by the bacteria to their reproductive organs. Pigs at all ages can become lame, arthritic, or develop an inflammation of the spinal column which leads to a paralysis of the hindquarters.

Sheep

Sheep are infected by *Brucella ovis,* a brucella bacteria specific to the species. Veneral infection takes place when diseased rams infect the ewes they are breeding by passing the bacteria in their semen. Clean rams are infected by ewes carrying microorganisms in their reproductive tracts that they acquired when previously serviced by a diseased ram. Infected ewes are brucella carriers but don't normally spread bacteria other than during breeding. Rams may remain actively infected and able to spread the disease for many years. They also infect each other by physical contact. There is a great difference in the number of infected rams at different ages: much fewer young males are diseased than older rams.

Rams become temporarily infertile because of the poor quality semen they produce when first infected. One or both of their testicles may become inflamed and will appear larger than normal when examined. The ewe's placenta becomes inflamed and she may abort or give birth to a dead lamb.

Goats

Goats are primarily infected by swallowing *Brucella melitensis* bacteria in their feed or drinking water. The brucellae pass into the bloodstream and concentrate and multiply in the udder and lymph glands. The most common symptom is abortion, usually occurring around the 4th month of pregnancy. If the fetus is carried to term, kids may be born dead or very weak and sickly. A vaginal discharge containing the bacteria continues for 2–3 weeks after abortion. Animals become infertile and are attacked by secondary bacterial invaders. They may develop mastitis, bronchitis, an inflammation of the cornea of the eye, become lame, and lose weight.

Horses

Horses infected with brucella bacteria (either *B. abortus* or *B. suis*) frequently develop an inflammation of the joints, muscles, or tendons, which, depending on its location in the body, is called *fistulous withers* (when the inflammation is located at the top of the back where the bottom of the neck begins), or *poll evil* (when the top of the head is inflamed). Small fluid-filled sacs containing brucellae form in these inflamed regions. The sacs swell and rupture, forming passages or ducts called *fistulas* in the affected tissue leading to the surface of the skin. After rupture of the sacs secondary bacterial infection begins. Once the fistulas reach the skin the pus and serumlike fluid that escape are a potential source of the spread of brucellosis to other animals, especially horses, cattle, and pigs.

In addition to these signs, mares infected with brucellae sometimes abort and are temporarily or permanently infertile. "Repeat breeders," as described for cows and sows, may result.

Control and Treatment Measures

Up until the present no effective and inexpensive brucellosis treatment has been developed for any animal species. Until practical treatments become available strict control measures are the only way to prevent infection by brucella bacteria. If a herd is suspected of having brucellosis each animal should be tested by your veterinarian and slaughtered should it react positively. "Test and slaughter" may sound like a drastic step but it is the only possible way to entirely eradicate the disease once and for all. Herds must be retested several times, removing and sending to slaughter those animals that react positively each time, until those that are left show negative reactions two to three tests in a row.

The most important control measure in cattle, rams, and goats (in countries where the disease is widespread) is vaccination at a young age. Calves are injected subcutaneously with 5 milliliters of a *Brucella abortus* vaccine named Strain 19, which increases their resistance to the disease. This vaccination doesn't rule out the possibility of infection in a severe outbreak, but greatly lowers the number of cases. As the calves mature they maintain the same amount of resistance to brucellosis as when they were first vaccinated.

New cattle that will be brought into your herd should be vaccinated or bought from herds that are clean of brucellosis and that react negatively when tested for the disease. Unvaccinated replacements, even though they test negatively, should be quarantined from the herd for at least 1 month for cattle and 3 months for pigs. At the end of this period they are tested again, and if they react negatively once more they are allowed to join the herd.

The only possible control of brucellosis in pigs is "test and slaughter," since no effective vaccine has been developed for them yet. Pigs that have been shown at agricultural fairs and that come in contact with other animals outside of their farm should be quarantined and tested before being allowed to return to their pen and herdmates. Sheep should be separated by age so that young animals are not infected by older ones. Brucellosis outbreaks are reduced if older rams and those with orchitis are culled and slaughtered, leaving the young breeding stock on the farm.

Leptospirosis

Leptospirosis is a contagious bacterial disease of horses, cattle, pigs, sheep, goats, and humans that produces many symptoms, ranging from fever and anemia to abortion and death. Infection is caused by microscopic, spiral-shaped leptospira bacteria with hooked ends that enter the animals' bodies in feed or water that has been contaminated with the urine of another animal that is diseased with leptospirosis. Bacteria may also penetrate the mucous membranes of the inner surface of the eyes, the vagina, nose, mouth, and through scrapes and wounds in the surface of the skin.

The leptospirae pass into the blood stream and are found in all body organs within a week. They collect in the kidneys and may be excreted in the urine of a diseased animal for years, infecting all susceptible, clean animals that they come in contact with. Physical contact with urine containing the bacteria or the ingestion of them are the two most common means of infection.

Symptoms

Cattle

Leptospirosis in cattle is often called by its common name, lepto, or is known as redwater in calves. The three bacterial varieties that cause the disease are *Leptospira pomona*, *L. grippotyphosa*, and *L. hardjo*.

Normally, when there is an outbreak of leptospirosis in a herd most, if not all, young calves become infected. Their body temperatures, measured rectally, rise quickly from a norm of 101.5°F [38.5°C] to 105°–106°F [40.5°–41°C], and they show signs of fever. Generally they lose their appetites, lie on the ground too weak to move with exhaustion, have difficulty breathing, are jaundiced, show blood in their urine, and because of the great loss of red blood cells, become anemic. The lost blood causes the urine to vary from a pink to a deep red, almost black color, and lasts for 2–3 days. As it ends, so too does the jaundice. Since the calf's body takes 1½–2 weeks to replace the red blood cells it has lost, the animal will be anemic during this period of recuperation. Of 20 calves in a herd infected with leptospirosis, 1 to 3 will die of the disease.

Heifers and mature cattle rarely show such noticeable signs of infection; this is especially true of dry cows and those that are attacked by *Leptospira hardjo*. On the other hand, the normal milk production of milk cows drops severely and the milk acquires the thick, yellowish look of old, heavy cream or colostrum, and may be streaked with blood. The udder may change from its normal firmness and become either soft and limp or else hard feeling, but it doesn't become inflamed. Slowly, over several weeks, the cow returns to its normal level of milk production. On the average, three-quarters of the adult cows in a herd become infected during the leptospirosis outbreak but rarely do any die.

Mature, pregnant cattle often abort 2–5 weeks after infection with leptospirae, and most commonly around the 7th month of pregnancy. Calves that are carried full term are born dead or weak, and the afterbirth and umbilical cord are frequently swollen and filled with the watery portion of the blood, the serum. Because disease symptoms are oftentimes not present or not seen in mature cattle, abortion in several cows at the same time may be the first warning that the herd is suffering from leptospirosis. However, cows that have aborted do not become infertile and their future pregnancies and births are usually normal.

Horses

Several leptospira bacteria cause abortion in mares and are suspected of being responsible for an intermittent disease of the eyes in horses and mules known by its scientific name, periodic ophthalmia, or, more commonly, moon blindness, which may eventually result in total blindness.

The first attack of moon blindness lasts 1–2 weeks, during which time, in the acute form, the horse's eyes tear, its eyelids go into spasms, the inner membrane lining of the eyelids becomes inflamed, as does the cornea, the horse is afraid of and avoids the light, its pupils contract, and pus seeps into the front part of the eyes. Subsequent attacks are common, each time causing more and more structural damage to the eyes; however, the length of time between each attack varies greatly. Before total blindness occurs a horse may develop cataracts, the optic nerve may degenerate, or the retina may detach from the rest of the eye.

During the original attack the horse shows a fever of 103°–105°F [39.5°–40.5°C], measured rectally, for several days. The animal becomes depressed, loses its appetite, and may have jaundice. The strange feature of leptospirosis in horses and mules is that abortion and the symptoms of periodic ophthalmia may not begin to occur until several years after the infection takes place. In less serious cases than the acute attack described above no symptoms may be observed at all. Some permanent damage may occur to the eyes, but you may never realize it until your horse walks into a tree or shows some other obvious sign of the impairment of its vision.

Pigs

Pigs are attacked by many types of leptospira: *L. pomona, L. grippotyphosa, L. canicola,* and *L. icterohemorrhagiae* to name a few. They often become diseased with leptospirosis through contact with wild animal urine, and serve as one of the most important sources of infection of many other animal species and humans because of the large number of bacteria they excrete.

Leptospira pomona is the most common cause of leptospirosis in pigs, but only a small number of animals show acute signs of disease in an infected group at any one time. Those that do have severe infections may be partially off feed or may lose their appetites completely, suffer from diarrhea, and show signs of fever for 1-3 days. The clearest sign you'll receive that your herd is diseased with lepto is when your pregnant gilts and sows abort or give birth to dead piglets late in their pregnancies.

Sheep and Goats

Because sheep and goats are range animals that are generally not raised and housed in intensive confinement operations, and since they do not have much contact with pigs, their incidence of leptospirosis is low. *L. pomona* is the cause of most of the cases of the disease that do occur, usually when sheep or goats are pastured or raised with infective cattle. The symptoms of disease are the same as those of cattle.

Control

Sanitation plays an important part in the control of leptospirosis because of the bacteria's need for moisture to survive. Standing water in puddles, low areas, wet fields, and swamps should be drained. Prevent the run-off of urine into these areas and ponds or streams. Animals should be fenced off from wet spots.

Since rats frequently infect farm animals, they should be eradicated on your farm. Pigs must be housed and raised away from cattle so as to not infect them. Leptospira cannot survive in dry conditions or where the pH is very high or very low—a point that should be considered when disinfecting housing.

When buying replacement animals for your herd you need to make sure that the herds these animals come from have passed blood serum tests for leptospirosis. A verbal guarantee isn't good enough; if the farmer or animal dealer you're buying from can't show you a certificate proving that his or her animals are leptospirosis-free, you don't want them no matter how cheap or good-looking they are. Cheap today may be very expensive tomorrow.

Even so, after satisfying yourself that the animals you've bought are free of lepto by examining their blood serum tests, treat them as if they were infected. All cattle and horses should get an intramuscular injection of streptomycin or dihydrostreptomycin once a day for up to 3 days (11 milligrams per pound of body weight). Small animals, such as pigs, sheep, and goats, get an intramuscular injection of streptomycin or dihydrostreptomycin once every 12 hours for up to 3 days (5-10 milligrams per pound of body weight).

The vaccination of all the cattle in your herd once a year with a leptospirosis bacterin will prevent abortions, stillbirths, and deaths, but so far has not been shown to prevent leptospira infections that locate in the kidneys. Vaccination will not prevent leptospirosis carrier animals from maintaining the bacteria in your herd, always threatening to infect susceptible herdmates. Gilts and sows must be vaccinated twice with leptospirosis bacterins before each breeding period to help them build the resistance to infection they will need during their pregnancies.

Treatment

Cattle

Leptospirosis must be considered a herd problem. As soon as the disease is diagnosed—usually by observing an abortion in a cow or heifer—vaccinate the whole herd and immediately begin treatment with the antibiotic dihydrostreptomycin. The injectin is given intramuscularly twice a day (5 milligrams per pound of body weight each time) according to your veterinarian's instructions. While the animals' bodies react to the vaccine by building antibodies, thereby developing active immunity, the antibiotic will kill leptospira bacteria that have already entered infected animals' systems and will protect those that are susceptible to attack.

Because of the public health danger posed by dihydrostreptomycin, milk may not be marketed or consumed for 4 days after ending treatment with the drug, nor may animals be sold for slaughter or their meat consumed for 1 month.

Horses

Specific leptospirosis treatments have not yet been developed for horses. Since there are multiple causes of periodic ophthalmia and because of the difficulty of determining what the true source of disease is, you should rely on your veterinarian to prescribe a treatment after a physical examination of your animal and the necessary laboratory tests.

Pigs

Pigs are treated very much like cattle. At the first sign of disease all animals are vaccinated with *Leptospira pomona* bacterin, and are injected intramuscularly every 12 hours with 5-10 milligrams per pound of body weight of streptomycin or dihydrostreptomycin. This will stop the abortions and will help animals develop a certain amount of immunity to infection for up to 6 months.

Sheep and Goats

Sheep and goats are also vaccinated with a bacterin—usually *L. pomona*—and are injected intramuscularly every 12 hours with 5-10 milligrams per pound of body weight of streptomycin or dihydrostreptomycin.

Listeriosis

Listeriosis is a bacterial disease, also called Listerellosis or circling disease, which may cause abortion or central nervous system injuries in many varieties of animals and humans. Of the domestic farm animals, sheep, goats, and cattle are the most severely affected; it is less of a problem in pigs, horses, and rabbits.

Infection

The disease is generally characterized by two different routes of infection, depending on the species and age of the animal. Adult sheep, goats, cattle, and horses most frequently show an inflammation of the brain or of the membrane surrounding the spinal column, which leads to serious central nervous system impairment. Listeriosis in young ruminants and pigs of all ages is normally a blood disease in which tissue of the liver is destroyed; in poultry it is also commonly a blood disease with injury to either the heart muscle or liver tissue.

Outbreaks usually take place in cold climates during cold weather. Warm regions of the world rarely experience the problem. Stress situations often set off the disease in susceptible animals. For example, a rash of infections may appear 2–4 days after a rapid drop in the temperature.

Ruminants confined in feedlots, especially sheep, often become infected by eating listeriosis-contaminated silage, and in particular, corn silage. The most important listeriosis-causing bacteria of ruminants, *L. monocytogenes,* thrives on the slightly alkaline environment created by fermented silage.

The bacteria are found in the soil, and are eaten by grazing and rooting animals along with the vegetation. As these animals defecate and their herdmates come in physical contact with the feces, they too swallow the microorganisms and become infected.

Symptoms

Sheep, Goats, and Cattle

Sheep and goats are the most rapidly and severely affected by listeriosis infection. Once they first show signs of disease they usually die within 4–48 hours. If they recover, and very few do, chances are good they will be left with at least some permanent central nervous system damage. The infection is slower and not as acute in cattle which normally show disease symptoms for 4 days to 2 weeks before dying.

Diseased animals separate themselves from their herdmates and lean up against walls, posts, fences, trees, and other fixed objects, trembling as if they would fall down otherwise. Occasionally they huddle in the corners of their pens or other housing. Animals will be seen walking in circles without varying the direction. This is the symptom that gives listeriosis its more commonly known name, circling disease.

Animals become feverish (lamb temperatures reach 106°F, and those of cattle vary between 104°–106°F [40°–41°C]), nervous, and lose their appetites completely. The mucous membranes of the inner lining of their eyelids often become inflamed and they sometimes go blind. In a visual examination you will notice that diseased animals either cannot control the muscles of their eyes, ears, and jaw in a normal fashion or that the muscles are totally paralyzed. Strands of saliva and mucus hang from their mouths and nostrils. They may become cross-eyed and their ears may hang down abnormally. The muscles of the front part of the body are stretched tighter and are held more rigidly than those of the hindquarters. The whole appearance of the sick animal is one of severe depression.

Before death, animals frequently lie on their sides and move their legs in a running motion. The whites of their eyes may turn gray and they pant rapidly.

Abortion or stillbirth may occur in late pregnancy in nanny goats, ewes, and cows. If so, the symptoms associated with brain inflammation—circling, facial paralysis, and so forth—are usually not seen at the same time within the herd. Oftentimes there are no apparent injuries to females when they abort, although they may have sustained some liver damage.

Pigs

Young pigs react more severely to listeriosis infection than older, more mature animals. Symptoms vary but are generally those seen with infection via the bloodstream and include fever, shaking, and trembling. They become restless, nervous, and their appetites are reduced. Pigs lose the normal control of their hind legs and may stagger stiffly on the front legs while they drag their hind legs behind them.

Young piglets go into spasms, become paralyzed (see Figure 75) and usually die within 4 days of the first well-established symptoms. Older animals are more resistant to listeriosis and recover more frequently from infection.

Poultry

Chickens, ducks, and geese are the most common domestic fowl that suffer from listeriosis, usually as a blood disease, but also occasionally in the central nervous system (CNS) form in which the brain becomes in-

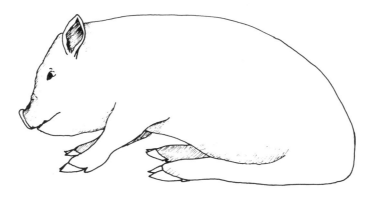

Figure 75.   A piglet with listeriosis showing paralysis of the hindquarters.

flamed. Generally young birds are more often diseased than older ones and, in the septicemic form, slowly lose condition before dying. Mature birds die quickly without showing any noticeable disease symptoms. In the CNS form birds suffer from wryneck, a condition in which the neck becomes twisted and the head is held to one side as a result of frequent contractions of the neck muscles. The skeletal muscles tremble and birds walk around in circles.

Poultry are believed to be among the major carriers of listeriosis, able to maintain infective bacteria within their bodies for years without ever showing signs of disease.

Control and Treatment

Most evidence seems to indicate that listeriosis infection takes place because of exposure to the disease-causing microorganisms in the environment (in soil, drinking water, pasture, and feed) and through contact with apparently healthy carrier animals. Carrier animals shed listeria bacteria in their feces, which when licked or swallowed by their healthy herdmates cause them to become infected. The disease also occurs because of stress conditions, including other diseases which weaken the animal's natural defenses.

Therefore, the animal's environment must be as sanitary and as healthful as possible. Feces and soiled bedding must be cleaned up regularly; housing and pens must be disinfected frequently, drinking water should be clean and plentiful; feed must be nutritious; parasites should be checked for and gotten rid of; vaccinations must be given at the right times and stress has to be constantly prevented.

No reliable vaccine for listeriosis has been developed yet for any animal species, nor has a specific drug been identified for treatment that gives a rapid and constant cure of the disease. Up to the time of the writing of this book the best drug results have come from the use of tetracyclines in high doses. Follow your veterinarian's advice as to the drug of choice. Despite some positive results with tetracyclines they have not always proved to work very well in CNS infections because of the difficulty of maintaining high enough concentrations in the brain tissue.

When the disease breaks out, those animals with proven cases of listeriosis must be separated from the rest of the herd. If you have been feeding silage you should immediately suspect it of being the source of infection. Send a sample to a laboratory for culture and discontinue feeding it for awhile to see what happens. When the pH of silage becomes acidic, as in the case of feed made from not entirely mature corn, silage becomes a less and less hospitable breeding ground for listeriae. Since spoiled silage has an alkaline pH, which the bacteria thrive on, never feed it to your animals.

A Caution about Identification and Human Infection

The symptoms of listeriosis are similar to those of other diseases in most animal species. As a result, diagnosis of the disease must be confirmed by a laboratory examination. In cattle, listeriosis may be mistaken for lead poisoning, thromboembolic encephalitis, an inflammation of the brain caused by a blood clot which blocks a blood vessel leading to the brain, polioencephalomalacia, a degeneration of the brain tissue caused by an inflammation of the nerve cells of the spinal cord, rabies, and brain abscesses. In sheep, listeriosis may be confused with brain abscesses, rabies, or pregnancy toxemia, a normally fatal blood sugar disease of ewes in late pregnancy caused by inadequate nutrition.

Listeria bacteria also cause several human diseases, the most common of which is miscarriage. Proper precautions must be taken when handling aborted animal fetuses and fetal fluids, and when doing autopsies of animals suspected of having died of listeriosis.

Tetanus

Tetanus is a CNS disease caused by a toxin produced by *Clostridium tetani* bacteria in most animals and humans when they receive deep puncture wounds or become infected during castrations, dockings, or during birth (via the umbilical cord). The disease, also called lockjaw because of one of its most apparent symptoms, is most common in horses, burros, mules, donkeys, and humans. It is very uncommon in poultry, which are quite resistant. Equines generally are infected through wounds in the feet; sheep also have a high incidence of tetanus and most often become diseased through unsterile dockings and castrations.

Tetanus occurs throughout the world, with the majority of cases located in regions with warm climates. In cases that aren't treated almost immediately after infection the probability of death is 80 percent or higher.

Infection

Clostridium tetani bacteria are anaerobic microorganisms (meaning they are only able to grow and multiply in the absence of air) that are commonly found in the soil of old farms, in heavily manured fields, in swamps, dust, hay, and manure. When they enter an animal's tissue, via a wound, along with a little bit of carrier material—soil, dust, manure, or the object that caused the wound in the first place—the damaged tissue dies and creates the proper environment for the bacteria to produce spores. When the dead tissue is broken down by enzymes, the spores contained within it release a powerful nerve toxin, which is absorbed by close-lying nerve tissue. The toxin, tetanospasmin, passes through the nerves until it reaches the spinal cord, where it causes the muscular contractions associated with the disease.

Symptoms

A week and a half to 2 weeks usually elapse between infection and the appearance of the first symptoms, but this incubation period may last as long as several weeks. The first signs that an animal shows are stiffness of the jaw or neck muscles (making chewing and swallowing slow and difficult), stiffening of the rear legs and the spot where it was wounded or infected. The next day the animal is stiff throughout its whole body. This is easily seen in the odd, stiff-legged way it moves, as if it were straddling something.

Muscular spasms are caused by the most inconsequential things: the movement of another animal or a shadow; any noise; a ray of light; being touched; a breeze. The head and neck are stretched up and forward by muscular contractions of the back and neck. As the spasms continue, walking, turning, or moving about become more difficult until the animal stops doing them altogether. The ears are held straight up as if listening intently to something, and the animal's tail sticks stiffly straight out behind it. In horses, the inner eyelid, which is usually not seen, emerges and covers part of the eyeball.

The animal is constipated and sweats, although its temperature is only a little above normal. Breathing and heart beat usually speed up and a white froth appears around the nostrils and mouth. Pigs, sheep, and goats frequently fall down and lie on their sides with both front and hind legs extended rigidly behind as far as they can go. Just before death the animal's temperature may rise quickly, reaching 108°–110°F (42°–43°C) (see Figure 76).

After the first symptoms are seen animals generally die within 1–2 weeks. On the average 20 percent of infected animals survive a tetanus infection, often taking 4–6 weeks to completely recover.

Control

In regions with high incidences of tetanus foals should receive injections of tetanus antitoxin starting at birth and every 2 weeks afterward until they are 3 months old, at which time they receive a tetanus toxoid injection. The antitoxin causes a passive resistance to disease, which protects the young animal until it is strong enough to develop active resistance from the toxoid injection. In areas where tetanus is not common or not a great risk foals should receive the toxoid when they are 5–8 weeks old.

Adult horses that haven't previously received toxoid vaccinations are injected with 1,500–3,000 International units (IUs) of antitoxin. Two weeks later they get another antitoxin shot and an injection of toxoid at the same time. One month after this the antitoxin and toxoid injections are repeated; then in the future they are given a toxoid booster once a year.

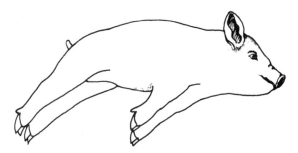

Figure 76. The rigid backwards extension of the legs is a typical tetanus symptom.

Mares get a toxoid shot in their final 6 weeks of pregnancy.

If tetanus is common in your area you should vaccinate sheep, goats, cows, and pigs. The method is similar to that in horses: start with the antitoxin, then 2 weeks later give both antitoxin and toxoid shots. This should be repeated in a few weeks. Pigs receive three series of the antitoxin and toxoid injections, each time leaving several weeks between vaccinations.

The prevention of tetanus is dependent on maintaining good sanitary controls, on preventing wounds, and on making sure wounds or surgical operations do not become contaminated with dirt or feces. Surgical instruments and needles must be sterilized repeatedly during even the simplest of operations, such as docking or castration. After the operation always use iodine to disinfect the wound. Animals have to be provided with clean, dry, dust-free, and disinfected pens in which to give birth. Their pens, stalls, enclosures, and pastures must be free of any sharp objects, waste materials, old pieces of metal, wires, nails, screws or cans—in short, anything on which they can injure themselves.

When castrations are done surgically, drainage of the wound needs to be complete. Animals should be placed on clean pasture, out of the sun, to recover. After birth, umbilical cords must be treated with an antiseptic, preferably iodine. Piglets should have their eyeteeth clipped soon after birth as they may injure each other or their sow, which could possibly permit the entry of *Cl. tetani* bacteria.

Treatment

Horses

Diseased horses can be saved if they are treated soon after infection; at later stages treatment is in vain. Give 300,000 IUs of tetanus antitoxin every 12 hours along with tranquilizers or sedatives to relax their muscles, according to your veterinarian's recommendation. The wound through which the horse became infected must be opened, cleaned thoroughly, and drained. Give an intramuscular injection of procaine penicillin G in an aqueous solution (5,000–10,000 IUs/lb of body weight once a day) or an intramuscular injection of tetracycline (1-5 mg/lb of body weight once a day).

The horse needs help to eat and drink without having to lower its head, so raise its feeder and waterer. If it can't get up or stay on its feet use a sling to support it. The stall should be dark, quiet, and filled with new, clean bedding. Pay close attention to your animal and respond quickly should it need help. Good nursing may pull it through.

Other Species

The treatment described above for horses is that generally recommended for other species: injection as soon after infection as possible with massive doses of tetanus antitoxin and penicillin or a broad spectrum antibiotic, and complete disinfection of the wound. The indicated drugs and dosages should be based on your veterinarian's suggestions. In spite of prompt treatment recovery is doubtful in sheep, goats, and pigs.

Mastitis: What Is It?

Mastitis is an inflammation of the mammary gland of a female animal that is commonly associated with cattle, but that occurs in most mammals as well. The inflammation may be directly caused by many types of bacteria and yeasts, which are allowed to enter the mammary gland by an injury, unsanitary milking conditions, improper or poorly functioning milking machinery, and faulty milking technique. More specifically this means that a cow steps on its udder while getting up or that if she has a heavy, low hanging udder, she bangs it on that old doorsill to the barn you've been meaning to replace. It could be that the vacuum pressure in the milking machine is too strong or too weak; perhaps you forgot to disinfect number 54's teats after milking her out; possibly, you were in a rush to get done with the evening milking so you didn't remember to disinfect your hands after finishing with each cow in the herd. The causes of mastitis are every bit as numerous as the cases are frequent.

Depending on its types and their severity the disease shows up in different forms, ranging from peracute to chronic to gangrenous.

Symptoms

Mastitis is a disease whose complicated and varied symptoms depend to a large extent on the specific infectious microorganism. The following descriptions are given in order to distinguish between the general forms the disease may take. See the next section, "Microorganisms that Cause Mastitis," for a further discussion of symptoms.

Peracute and Acute Mastitis

These two forms are only differentiated by the degree of the animal's reaction to infection. A peracute is a more intense or pronounced response than an acute infection.

Cows (as well as mares, ewes, nanny goats, and sows) become ill quickly. They might appear fine during the morning milking but show clear signs that something is seriously wrong by evening milking. The animal appears depressed; she's off feed partially, or completely loses her appetite; her eyes are sunken, and her pulse is weaker and faster than the normal 60–70 heart beats per minute. The cow's temperature goes to 103°F or higher from its usual 99.5°–102°F [38°–39°C] and it looks feverish.

The udder is hot, swollen, and painful in one or more quarters. This may be how you first realize something is wrong, especially if an old, calm, and usually easy-going cow tries to jump through the roof when you wash her down prior to milking her. If she doesn't put you into orbit with a well-placed kick, you'll quickly realize that you have a problem when you milk her out because her production will be way down. In addition, the milk will look strange. Depending on the attacking bacteria the milk may be watery with yellow, buttery clots or so watery that it is hard to believe that it's milk at all. It can have a stringy, mucuslike feel to it, or be regular old milk but filled with off-color specks. Whichever it is, you know the cow has mastitis and you had better do something about it rapidly before it gets worse or spreads through the herd.

These types of the disease are frequently caused by a stressful incident. It could have been a kick from another animal, a cold snap that the animal's body defenses weren't prepared for, a bee sting on the teat or udder, a cut with barbed wire, and so on.

Chronic Mastitis

Chronic mastitis is seen in cows that get a milder case of the disease than described above. They are treated and apparently cured. Then 3 months later or in their next lactation they get mastitis again; and this happens over and over again.

It's not certain that these animals will show outward signs of disease, but what is unmistakeable is that their milk will look abnormal (it could be flecked, clotted, or cheesy). Be sure to examine the strip cup, the small cup that milk from each of a cow's quarters is milked into, before milking her out, to check for abnormalities and disease. Oftentimes, this milk will not pass through the strainer into the bulk tank.

Gangrenous Mastitis

Gangrenous mastitis may occur after a peracute or acute infection, or without any warning at all. When one or more of the teats or quarters begins to feel hard and cold, like the skin of a reptile, and turns blue, you know your cow has gangrenous mastitis. The skin feels dead for a good reason—it is!

Usually the gangrene is caused by the swelling produced in response to the mastitis infection. The swelling cuts off the blood supply to the udder tissue and it begins to die. The dead tissue rots and decays, releasing toxins that are rapidly carried throughout the cow's body. The next thing you know you've got a dead, foul-smelling animal on your hands. If a cow isn't treated very quickly after its udder starts to feel cold chances are good it will die.

Microorganisms that Cause Mastitis

Staphylococci Bacteria

Staphylococcus aureus is a round-shaped bacteria which causes most of the mastitis in cattle. It enters the animal through any wound or sore of the skin, teats, and udder, and has developed a strong resistance to penicillin, the main antibiotic which had been used to kill it.

It has been found that in herds that repeatedly suffer from staphylococci mastitis outbreaks, generally more than half of the cattle have infections whose symptoms are too mild to be observed by the farmer and are only diagnosed as diseased by testing (see "A Quick Test for Mastitis," p. 193). *St. aureus* causes all of the different forms of disease mentioned previously. Dry cows, those that the farmer has stopped milking prior to their having a calf, with unapparent (subclinical) infections are cured more easily than those that are being milked. If an animal remains infected for over a year it is likely that treatment won't work.

Streptococci Bacteria

Streptococcus agalactiae, the main streptococci bacteria that causes mastitis in cattle, must live within the udder to survive. These microorganisms enter the teats through their openings and multiply quickly in the milk and on the walls of the ducts that carry the milk secreted by the udder. They damage the milk-secreting tissue of the duct walls and cause the ducts to get plugged up with loose and broken up cells and wastes. This stimulates a greater than normal production of fibrous tissue to hold the cells together. As a result the udder is no longer able to secrete milk in this area.

Cows are infected during milking. Typically, in spite of disinfection of the udder and milking machine, the bacteria are spread from one animal to another via infected milk. Calves infect each other by consuming milk containing streptococci from one of the mature, diseased cows in the herd and then by sucking each other's teats.

Other streptococci that are able to survive outside of the udder and that also cause mastitis are *Str. uberis, Str. dysgalactiae, Str. zooepidemicus,* and others. The first two are normal problems on dairy farms; *Str. zooepidemicus* more frequently affects mares and sows but can be passed to cattle on farms where different animal species are pastured or housed together.

Coliform Bacteria

Milk normally contains white blood cells which combat infection by harmful bacteria. When these white blood cells are at low levels and a coliform infection takes place, the injurious bacteria are able to multiply very rapidly. The animal's body reacts to the infection with an inflammation that kills the attacking microorganisms. But ironically, this is when the real danger begins because as the coliform bacteria die they release endotoxins, poisonous protoplasm, which cause a peracute mastitis.

Coliform infections are most commonly caused by the rod-shaped bacteria, *Escherichia coli* (more popularly known as *E. coli*), *Aerobacter aerogenes,* and the *Klebsiellas.*

Infected animals show the classic signs of peracute infection: depression, diarrhea, loss of appetite, loss of weight, and dehydration. The cow has a high fever that ranges between 103°–108°F [39°–42°C] and milk production stops altogether, but not before a brown, watery fluid is seen in the milk. When the attacking bacteria is a *Klebsiella,* animals often swell up in the joints, and, most particularly in the hocks.

Cattle with low white blood cell levels in their milk, and older animals whose teat openings are looser than those of younger animals, are most often infected with coliform mastitis.

Gilts and sows frequently get peracute infections 1-2 days after farrowing. They become weak, have no energy, and neglect their piglets. Water and food intake drop off or stop outright. Temperatures are a little higher than normal and may reach 107.6°F [42°C]. The teats and udder become painfully swollen and purple, and the milk they produce is the watery-creamy consistency of serous fluid or pus. Blood clots or a fibrous material that forms when blood coagulates may be seen.

Piglets will look hungry and thin. They try to nurse frequently and go back and forth from nipple to nipple. Since they are unsatisfied with the short periods the sow lets them nurse, if she does at all, they wander about the pen trying to satiate their hunger by nosing at and chewing litter and licking urine instead of lying in a heap with their littermates.

In bad cases animals are stiff and become disoriented and dizzy. They remain motionless, lying on their stomachs, and may go into comatose states. If this continues death ensues.

A Quick Test for Mastitis

The California Mastitis Test (CMT) is a kit that contains a plastic paddle with little hollows in it and several bottles of chemicals used to test for mastitis. Milk samples are mixed in the hollows with different chemicals by carefully moving the paddle in a circular motion while holding it horizontal to the ground.

Based on the amount of material that settles out of the milk/chemical mixture you can estimate how inflamed a cow's quarter is. If nothing settles out your cow doesn't have mastitis or is not shedding the infectious bacteria in its milk at the present time (in the case of a chronic carrier animal). If any abnormal looking material should settle out call your veterinarian in to take samples to determine what the attacking microorganism is in order to begin treatment. The CMT should be done once a month on all lactating cows and whenever you have reason to suspect mastitis in your herd.

Control Measures

With mastitis, as with many diseases, control should start with a hard look at management practices. Since we know that *Str. agalactiae* doesn't survive out of the udder, its spread in a herd is most likely due to milking technique.

Do you wear rubber gloves and disinfect your hands after milking out one cow and before going to the next? Do you always dip all of your cows' teats in a chlorine, clorhexidine, or iodine solution after you have milked them? Before milking do you wash a cow's teats and udder with warm, running water and an antiseptic soap solution? Do you use individual paper towels to dry the udder, and then throw them away? These are the types of questions we need to ask ourselves.

Additionally, make sure your milking machine works properly. Check the vacuum level, pressure, and pulsation rate; the milk liners must not be too wide (less than 1 inch is best) and the vacuum must be released as soon as the cow milks out.

Before milking always hand strip a little bit of milk from each quarter into a strip cup in order to do a quick visual check for mastitis or other abnormal conditions. Disinfect your hands each time and dispose of this milk. Don't add it to the bulk tank.

To prevent the spread of mastitis within the herd milk heifers that test negatively on the CMT first, then clean cows, followed by those animals that have recently had mastitis and that have been treated for it, and finally, cows and heifers that have tested positively on the CMT and that currently suffer from mastitis. This way you won't accidentally infect a clean cow with mastitis if there should be a momentary lapse in the other management safeguards. Likewise, don't allow clean cows to lie where infected cows do, or mastitis-causing bacteria will be transmitted in the little bit of milk that leaks out of the diseased cow's teats before milking. This is a consideration in older, high producing cows that begin to let their milk down in anticipation of milking or whose sphincter muscles (the muscle that encircles the inside of the teat openings) are loose.

All cuts, scrapes, sores, cracking, or chapping of the teats or udder should be washed, disinfected, and treated with an antiseptic salve or ointment until they heal. These are possible points of entry for the bacteria that cause mastitis.

All replacement heifers and cows must receive the CMT and have their milk samples cultured by a laboratory, with negative results, before being allowed to enter the milking herd. Never feed milk from cows with suspected or confirmed cases of mastitis to calves, and don't let the calves suck each other's teats. Any cows that come down repeatedly with mastitis should be gotten rid of. Strict culling is an important control measure and will help keep your money where it should be—in your pocket—and not in continual and expensive treatments.

Sows should be held in well disinfected, individual farrowing pens starting a few days before they have their litters and continuing until the piglets are weaned.

Treatment

Mastitis treatments are as complicated as the disease is itself. Conventional wisdom has it that peracute and acute mastitis should be treated simultaneously with an intramuscular systemic injection and an intramammary infusion of the antibiotic that is specific to the bacteria causing the infection. However, the usefulness of intramammary infusion (done with a "mastitis tube" filled with an antibiotic that is introduced into the teat canal and whose contents are expelled into the quarter) has recently been called into question by farmers and veterinarians alike who feel its potential benefits may be outweighed by its drawbacks.

The inside of a cow's udder looks like the cross-section of a natural sponge: the tissue is arranged in an apparently miscellaneous pattern with tiny ducts and channels meandering throughout the gland. When mastitis-causing microorganisms attack the tissue of one or more quarters they disrupt and destroy, depending on the severity of the infection, the normal milk secretion which takes place on the interior surface of the udder tissue. Oftentimes, especially in chronically infected animals, the udder reacts to the destruction of its spongelike tissue by developing a new layer of tissue which surrounds and cuts off the injured tissue. This barrier can prevent the antibiotic ointment or suspension that has been infused into the udder with a "mastitis tube" from reaching the infectious bacteria. And even though we attempt to maintain antiseptic conditions while we give the infusion, by disinfecting the udder, the teat, the teat opening, the "mastitis tube," and our hands, it is impossible to completely prevent the introduction of more, and possibly harmful, bacteria into the teat canal and udder.

For these reasons there will be a continuing discussion of the benefits and disadvantages of intramammary infusion. I feel that systematic treatment is effective and needs no additional support, except in very serious infections. But since there is no widely accepted consensus on which treatment is best, both are included in the following section, "Mastitis Treatment Guide for Cattle." Check with your veterinarian on this and watch farming journals for further developments.

Systemic injection and intramammary infusion are done once a day for 3-4 days. Keep the mastitis-infected cow in the barn, separated from its herdmates, and keep milking her out every few hours during the day. What you are trying to do is flush out the infective bacteria. *Don't use this milk!* Make sure it is disposed of where other animals can't get to it. Pay very close attention to the warnings on the bottle or packaging the antibiotic comes in since the drug will pass into the milk for different lengths of time depending on the specific product and it should not be used for human consumption.

Generally, subclinical infections are treated for when cows are dried off because they respond better than when lactating. The udder is infused with an antibiotic solution that lasts a long time. A cow that was treated for a subclinical case of mastitis when dried off that has a new flare-up after freshening (giving birth) is a prime candidate for culling from the herd as soon as you can manage it.

Since peracute and acute mastitis in sows are usually caused by coliform bacteria, we will limit our discussion of treatment to this group. Peracute cases can be treated with an intramuscular injection of oxytetracycline (3-5 mg/lb of body weight once daily until recovery), dihydrostreptomycin (5-10 mg/lb of body weight once to twice a day until 1 day after the sow looks all right), or ampicillin (check with your veterinarian for dosage). Trimethoprim with sulfamethoxazole, polymyxin, neomycin, chloramphenicol, and gentamycin may also be used. The sow's udders should be massaged with warm towels or by hand and repeatedly stripped out. Put an udder ointment or salve that contains menthol or some other ingredient that has a heat-producing effect on the affected udder.

Piglets should be given a milk substitute or fostered onto another lactating sow or they will starve to death. Sweet condensed milk is mixed half and half with boiled water (after it has cooled to lukewarm) and fed in a baby bottle if the piglets are strong enough to suck. If they are too weak to suck give them an intraperitoneal injection of electrolytes and 15 ml of a sterile 5 percent glucose solution. Then get some milk mixture into their bellies by squeezing a little at a time down their throats with an eyedropper. They will have to swallow to keep from choking. Make sure you don't overfeed them. Repeat the glucose injection a few hours later. Be sure that all piglets that have been fed are under the heat lamp, huddled together, and sleeping as a group. It is important to prevent them from catching cold in their weakened state.

Goats should be treated systemically in the same way cows are and are milked out frequently. Check with your veterinarian for a recommended broad spectrum antibiotic. Always culture a milk sample to determine what the attacking microorganism is and how to treat for it. If coliform mastitis is suspected (because of a cold, dead-feeling quarter) immediately give a cortisone shot to bring down the swelling. Next give an intramuscular injection of a broad spectrum antibiotic and apply hot compresses to the udder. In Great Britain herbal remedies for mastitis treatment in goats have achieved considerable success. One of them, a tea made by boiling dock and elder, is used to massage the udder. Put a handful of both dock and elder into an enamel pot and pour in boiling water. Cover the pot and let it steep overnight. At the next morning's milking soak a cloth in the tea and massage the goat's udder. Make a new tea each day and use it to massage the whole udder each time you milk the goat. If you can't find dock or elder, try wood sage.

Mastitis in the female rabbit is usually caused by an attack of staphylococci or streptococci. The nipples and mammary gland become inflamed, red looking, and hot to the touch. Give does an intramuscular injection of procaine penicillin G in an aqueous solution (10,000–20,000 units/lb of body weight once a day). Your veterinarian may have further recommendations.

Mastitis Treatment Guide for Cattle

Since so many different microorganisms cause so many different types of mastitis, I have summarized the main ones and their treatments into the following table. As you will notice from the title, the guide is only intended for use with cattle; the treatment of other species is briefly discussed in the preceding section, "Treatment."

The guide is divided into the following columns: Mastitis Causing Microorganisms, Type of Infection, Treatment, and Other Information. Mastitis Causing Microorganisms is self-explanatory. Type of Infection refers to the seriousness and form of the outbreak: for example, peracute, acute, subclinical, and so on. The Treatment column recommends which drug to use, at which dosage, for how long. The column headed Other Information suggests different drugs which may be used for treatment and related information, such as the means of infection.

This guide must be used based on your experience and that of your veterinarian. Drug treatments change frequently as microorganisms develop resistance, as more germ specific drugs are placed on the market, and as more is learned of the mechanisms of mastitis infection. Your veterinarian, the farm journals you read, and your state or region's agricultural university's extension service are good sources of information about what new developments are taking place in mastitis therapy. It is to your economic advantage to stay abreast of the changes in treatment.

Pasteurellosis

Pasteurellosis will probably always be called shipping fever, the common name by which it is known. Nevertheless, the term shipping fever is not entirely accurate, animals don't have to be shipped to come down with this infectious bacterial disease. What is required is stress and initial exposure to a virus and then to pasteurellae bacteria, all of which are encountered by animals being transported.

Depending on the animal species, pasteurellosis manifests itself throughout the world as either pneumonia, an inflammation of the lungs, or septicemia, blood poisoning. Cattle, sheep, pigs, goats, and rabbits are infected with the pneumonia form; septicemia affects sheep, pigs, and rabbits.

Mastitis Causing Microorganism	Type of Infection	Treatment	Other Information
Staphylococci Bacteria (*Staphylococcus aureus*)	Peracute and acute	a. *Systemic:* The following drugs may be used 1. Dihydrostreptomycin injected intramuscularly (5–10 mg/lb of body wt) 1–2 times per day. Continue treatment until 1 day after cow looks normal 2. Chlortetracycline injected intravenously twice a day (1–2.5 mg/lb of body wt). Continue treatment until cow's temperature is normal for 1 day 3. Erythromycin in a 200 mg/ml solution, injected intravenously every 12 hours (1–2 mg/lb of body wt). Continue treatment until 1 day after cow looks normal b. *Intramammary Infusion:* Laboratory culture will indicate which of the following drugs will be most effective 1. Erythromycin infusion given after milking in the morning, the evening, and the following morning (300 mg each time) 2. Chlortetracycline ointment given into the teat canal (400 mg). Give again 1–2 days later until cow is cured 3. Neomycin ointment given into the teat canal (500 mg). Give again 1–2 days later if cow doesn't look normal 4. Lincomycin Hydrochloride infusion (200 mg at a time) given 3 times every 12–24 hrs 5. Sodium Cloxacillin in a 3% Aluminum Monostearate base infused into the diseased quarter. Give (200 mg at a time) every 2 days for 6 days c. *Intramammary Infusion for Dry Cows Only* 1. Give an infusion of procaine penicillin G (1 million units) mixed with dihydrostreptomycin (1 g)	5. Milk cow normally (twice a day) 1. Give infusion after cow has been milked for the last time. Don't

Mastitis Causing Microorganism	Type of Infection	Treatment	Other Information
	Subclinical	a. *Intramammary Infusion for Dry Cows Only* 1. Benzathine cloxacillin in a 3% aluminum monostearate base (give 500 mg in total). Infused into all quarters 2. Give an infusion of procaine penicillin G (1 million units) mixed with dihydrostreptomycin (1 g)	give the infusion 2 weeks before calving up until birth 1. Don't milk out 2. Give infusion after cow has been milked for last time. Don't give the infusion 2 weeks before calving
Streptococci Bacteria (*Streptococcus Agalactiae; Str. uberis; Str. dysgalactiae; Str. zooepidemicus*)	All types	a. *Intramammary Infusion* Any of the following drugs may be used. 1. Penicillin (100,000 units) and dihydrostreptomycin sulfate (1 g) in an emulsion are infused into the teat canal once a day for 4 days 2. Oxytetracycline ointment (200–400 mg) is infused into the teat canal of the infected quarter. Give again 1–2 days later if cow doesn't look normal 3. Sodium cloxacillin in a 3% aluminum monostearate base is infused into the diseased quarter. Give (200 mg at a time) every 2 days for 6 days 4. Chlortetracycline ointment is infused into the teat canal (400 mg) Give again 1–2 days later until cow is cured b. *Intramammary Infusion for Dry Cows Only* Any of the following drugs may be used. 1. A procaine penicillin G infusion (300 mg) is	1. This penicillin-dihydro-streptomycin emulsion is specific to *Str. Agalactiae.* The other streptococci may be resistant to it 3. Milk cow normally (twice a day)

Organism	Type	Treatment	Notes
		given into each quarter when the cow is dried off 2. Benzathine cloxacillin in a 3% aluminum mosostearate base (500 mg in total) is infused into all quarters when the cow is dried off 3. A mixture of procaine penicillin G. (300 mg) and novobiocin (250 mg) in a base solution is infused into all quarters when the cow is dried off	2. Don't milk out
Coliform Bacteria (*E. coli; Aerobacter aerogenes; Klebsiella*)	Peracute and acute	a. *Systemic Injection and Intramammary Infusion:* 1. Dihydrostreptomycin injected intramuscularly (5–10 mg/lb body wt) 1–2 times per day. Continue treatment until 1 day after cow looks normal. Also give an intramammary infusion of dihydrostreptomycin (1–5 g) in an aqueous solution	1. Oxytetracycline, neomycin, and chlortetracycline can be substituted but aren't as reliable
	Subclinical	a. *Intramammary Infusion:* 1. Dihydrostreptomycin sulfate (0.25–1 g) in an oil-in-water suspension is infused into the teat canal. Give again in 1-½ days until milk tests normally again	
Pseudomonas aeruginosa	All types	a. *Intramammary Infusion* 1. Sodium carbenicillin infused into the teat canal of the diseased quarter (5 g each time) given once a day for 2 days, with 24 hours between each infusion	1. Check with your veterinarian for other drugs that may give better results and what systematic treatment he or she recommends for a peracute infection
Corynebacterium pyogenes	Peracute and acute	a. *Systemic Injection and Intramammary Infusion:* 1. Penicillin ointment or suspension (containing 100,000 units) infused into teat canal once a day for 2 days, with 24 hours between each infusion. Consult with your veterinarian for	1. Milk out twice a day

Mastitis Causing Microorganism	Type of Infection	Treatment	Other Information
	Subclinical and for dry cows	the recommended penicillin dose of the simultaneous intramuscular injection a. *Intramammary Infusion:* 1. Procaine penicillin G in a slow-releasing base (300 mg) is infused into each quarter twice when the cow is dried off and midway into its dry period	1. This drug mixture may be known by the brand name of Altapen
	Many abscesses of the udder	Slaughter	
	All types except subclinical	Slaughter	
Nocardia asteroides	Subclinical	*Intramammary Infusion:* 1. A furaltadone and penicillin mixture is infused into the teat canal every 12 hours for at least 1-½ days or until the milk culture is normal	
Mycoplasma	All types	Slaughter	1. Mycoplasma mastitis has occurred in England, Canada, the U.S, Australia, and Israel
Yeast	All types	1. Stop penicillin or other antibiotic treatment 2. Consult with your veterinarian	1. Yeasts in the udder multiply when antibiotics are used 2. Outbreaks may occur when attempting to treat *Streptococcus agalactiae*

Symptoms

Cattle

Cattle develop pasteurellosis as a result of many kinds of stress. Stressful conditions include shipping, abrupt temperature changes, overcrowding, too warm and damp a barn, lengthy periods without food or water, a change in the diet, excitement, very dusty conditions, and exhaustion. Recently weaned calves are most susceptible to these kinds of stress.

Infected cows lose their appetites, their milk production drops, they become thin and depressed, and develop a fever that ranges from 104°-108°F (41°-42°C), well above their normal body temperature of 100.5°-102.5°F (38°-39°C). A watery discharge is seen from the nostrils and sometimes the eyes. The pulse speeds up from the normal 60-70 beats per minute. The breathing of a sick cow is quick and shallow, almost a pant. The lungs make a wet, spitting sound or else sound as if the tissue is rubbing on itself inside. Later in the course of the disease these sounds from the lungs decrease and may stop altogether. The animal shows obvious signs of breathing problems: it holds its neck stretched forward, its nostrils are spread as wide as they can go, and it may grunt with each breath. After starting to grunt, cows usually die quickly.

Sheep

In mild infections of the pneumonia-causing pasteurellae sheep cough and have a watery discharge from the nostril and eyes. They look dazed, are off feed, and have difficulty breathing. Their temperatures rise above normal from a usual 103°F (39°C) to up to 107°F (41.5°C). In acute attacks animals will die quickly without much warning. This same pasteurella strain causes a septicemic infection, as well as pneumonia, in lambs that are less than 2 months old.

Sheep that become infected with the septicemic type of pasteurellosis generally show symptoms of disease after their diet has been suddenly improved. The causes are numerous: they have been moved to lush leguminous pasture or they may have been started on a heavy grain ration without any buildup. A few days after this feeding change, sheep, and particularly those of about 6 months of age, begin to look dazed and depressed. They stay in one place and don't want to move, their breathing is difficult, and foam drips from their mouths. Temperatures are higher than normal until shortly before death. Paradoxically, healthy looking sheep die first; up to one-fifth of a flock may die over a few days once the septicemic outbreak begins.

Pigs

It is generally accepted that pigs become diseased with pasteurellae during periods when their normal respiratory defenses are weak. They breathe in the bacteria in droplets or mists which are coughed out or respired by infected herdmates. Pasteurellae must quickly find their preferred environment—a weakened respiratory system—after being shed by an infected pig because they are only able to live a few weeks out of the animal and are killed by direct sunlight in 10 minutes.

Pigs with pasteurellosis usually show classic signs of peneumonia: they start with a dry cough that quickly turns wet as the lungs fill with a foamy liquid. Breathing becomes difficult and a "thumping" sound is heard with each breath. Animals go off feed, lose weight and condition, are depressed, and appear weak. In acute attacks (these usually last 5-10 days) temperatures may go to 105°-107°F (40.5-41.5°C), well above the normal 101°-103°F [38°-39.5°C] range. Animals with acute infections commonly die if not treated, but the chronic form is seen more often.

An acute septicemic pasteurellosis also occurs. Animals have difficulty breathing (the throat becomes swollen), they become very depressed, stop eating and may collapse. Temperatures shoot up very high to 105°-108°F (40.5°-42°C) and the skin may look bluish-red. Pigs may start dying a few hours after the first signs are noticed or they may survive up to a week longer.

Rabbits

Pasteurellae cause all sorts of different problems in rabbits: snuffles, an inflammation of the mucous membranes of the lungs and nasal passages, abscesses anywhere in the body, an infection of the reproductive tract, and pneumonia.

In snuffles a thin pus drips from the eyes and nostrils. Rabbits paw at and rub their noses with their front paws, and sneeze, shake their heads, and cough. The reproductive infection is characterized by a heavy yellow-gray pus flowing from the vagina of the doe and dripping from the penis of the buck. Commonly, one or both of the buck's testicles are swollen. If one of the doe's uterine horns is infected she can conceive young in the other; if both are infected she is normally incapable of bearing young.

Rabbits with pneumonia are weak, sleeply looking, lose their appetites, have diarrhea, and difficulty breathing. Their temperatures go to 104°F [40°C], and if they are not treated, they die in several days.

Control Measures

Cattle

A reduction of stressful conditions goes a long way toward controlling shipping fever. Keep animals that have been shipped isolated from the rest of the herd while you observe and treat them if necessary.

Veterinarians are split down the middle as to the pros and cons of vaccination. Some say that pasteurellosis antiserum is God's gift to the world, others will tell you just as emphatically that the antiserum has no effect whatsoever. The battle has been raging for years and shows no signs of letting up or of coming to any definite conclusion.

Sheep

The same controversy exists over theories for the treatment of sheep. Probably the best general control measure is once again the reduction and elimination of stress. Sheep should have their diets changed slowly, with a gradual increase in their nutritional levels. New feeds are fine, but they should be introduced gradually.

Pigs

Don't allow pigs to come down with respiratory infections. Since pasteurellae are secondary bacterial invaders, they need weakened respiratory defenses to be able to gain a foothold in the lungs and to multiply. Don't give them the chance.

Specific pathogen-free herds or closely controlled closed herds, ones into which no outside animals are introduced for either breeding or replacement, offer hope in the reduction of the infections which predispose animals to infection by pasteurellae. Vaccination with pasteurella bacterin looks promising and should be investigated with your veterinarian. Stress reduction and good management practices are the most important controls you can institute.

Rabbits

Rabbits develop pasteurellosis when their resistance to disease is low, when they are subjected to stress (scanty or wet bedding, drafts, poor sanitation, unbalanced rations, and so on) or when kindling—giving birth. Pay attention to the basics: good management, elimination of stress, and prevention of other diseases, especially enteritis (inflammation of the intestines), which enables pasteurellae to infect rabbits as secondary invaders.

Treatment

Cattle

Once pasteurellosis or any pneumonialike symptoms are observed call your veterinarian and have him or her examine the infected animal. In addition to prescribing a drug treatment it is likely they will recommend some supportive therapy to decongest the animal's lungs. These treatments may make all the difference in getting your cow back in production quickly and in preventing the spread of the disease through the herd.

Separate diseased cattle from their herdmates as soon as symptoms are noted. If pasteurellosis is diagnosed shortly after infection, inject animals intramuscularly twice or three times a day with a combination of procaine penicillin G in an aqueous suspension and dihydrostreptomycin in an aqueous suspension until their body temperatures and breathing return to normal and they begin eating again for one full day. Each cow should receive a total of 5,000–10,000 units/lb of the body weight of procaine penicillin G and 5–10 mg/lb of body weight of dihydrostreptomycin per day. Remember to divide these dosages into two (given every 12 hours) or three (given every 8 hours) equal-sized injections.

If the disease is to be treated at a later stage give an intravenous or intramuscular injection of oxytetracycline (5 mg/lb of the body weight once a day for 3 days) or an intravenous or intraperitoneal injection or oral dose of sulfamethazine (91 mg/lb of body weight once a day for 3 days). If you can't find either of these drugs, any broad spectrum antibiotic or sulfanamide specific for pasteurellosis may be substituted. Check with your veterinarian for the exact dosage.

It really doesn't matter with which drug you begin treatment but once you start out with one medication stick with it through the whole course of treatment, which usually lasts 3-4 days. If you change drugs half way through the treatment or only give a couple of shots and then stop, the cow may relapse (become ill again), the infectious micro-organisms may become resistant to the drug you used, and recuperation may take longer.

Sheep

As with cattle, your veterinarian should be called in to examine sheep with pasteurellosis or pneumonialike symptoms. Diseased animals are separated from the rest of the flock and their herdmates' temperatures are taken to determine if they were infected. Animals with temperatures over 103°F (39.5°C) are assumed to be diseased and should be treated. Keep a close watch on the rest of the flock and separate and treat any animals with disease symptoms over the next few days.

If the disease takes the form of pneumonia—coughing, a discharge from the eyes and nostrils, heavy breathing, and so forth—give an intra-muscular or intravenous injection of oxytetracycline (1-3 mg/lb of body weight) once a day until 1 day after the animal has returned to normal. Try to keep diseased sheep eating by offering them tidbits of cut-up vege-tables, apples, or bread. If the disease takes the septicemic form treat-ment is normally uncertain because of the rapidity and severity of in-fection. Ask your veterinarian's advice about treatment.

Pigs

Diseased pigs are separated from their penmates and held in dry sickbay pens that contain new, clean bedding. Treatment should begin at once with one of the following broad-spectrum antibiotics: chloram-phenicol, gentamycin, or ampicillin. In general, pasteurellae bacteria are becoming fairly resistant to penicillin, tetracycline, streptomycin, and sulfamethoxydin. Check with your veterinarian for the recom-mended drug and dosage.

Rabbits

Diseased rabbits are moved to their own clean and dry, well-bedded hutches, away from healthy rabbits. Any of the following drugs may be used for treatment as soon as disease symptoms are noted: oxytetra-cycline given as an intramuscular injection in equal doses every 6 hours (1.25 mg/lb of body weight for each injection) or every 12 hours (2.5 mg/lb of body weight for each injection); procaine penicillin G given as an intramuscular injection (10,000-20,000 units/lb of body weight once a day); or chlortetracycline given orally in equal doses every 6 hours (3.75-12.5 mg/lb of body weight) or every 12 hours (7.5-25 mg/lb of body weight).

Anemia: What Is It?

Blood circulates in the animal's body, just as it does in ours, carrying food and oxygen to all parts and removing waste products. Two main constituents of blood are red blood cells and white blood cells. White blood cells fight infection and diseases. Red blood cells combine with oxygen in the lungs and then supply the oxygen to the different parts of the body. They are both constantly being made and destroyed during the entire life of the animal.

The most important component of the red blood cells is hemoglobin. Hemoglobin is a combination of protein and iron which actually takes up the oxygen from the lungs. Copper and cobalt aid in the formation of red blood cells, and therefore of hemoglobin, but they don't become part of either one.

If the animal doesn't receive enough iron, copper, or cobalt two things can happen: not enough red blood cells are made to replace the ones that have died, or the new red blood cells don't contain enough hemoglobin. Either problem is called anemia.

Warning Signs

Because anemic animals lose their appetites they become pale, weak, and thin, sometimes they show a rapid pulse and shortness of breath. In other cases they have trouble breathing after any kind of exercise such as running, a condition called thumps (because of the sound they make). The animal grows poorly and takes longer than normal to develop sexually. Anemia usually occurs in young animals and most often when they're from 1-6 weeks old.

Anemic pigs sometimes swell up in the head and shoulders and often go into shock after receiving a vaccination against hog cholera. In general, anemic animals will be depressed and without strength. They may also have either diarrhea or constipation.

Prevention

The best prevention against anemia in cattle, sheep, goats, horses, donkeys, and mules is to feed them a mineralized salt that contains iron, cobalt, and copper. Premature or twin calves, whose level of nutrition is low (this can be determined from both their condition and the cow's condition) should receive an iron shot within their first week. They receive 6 cubic centimeters (6 cm³) of iron solution intramuscularly in either the neck or thigh muscle. Piglets should receive an iron injection as well. The best results occur if the injection is given when they are a few days old but it is of value up to 6 weeks. See the next section, "Anemia Prevention in Piglets."

Anemia, which is usually a nutritional disease, can also be caused by hemorrhage (loss of a large quantity of blood) and by ticks, lice, and parasites that suck the animal's blood. Certain parasites destroy red blood cells as well. For this reason animals should be purged on a regular basis and checked frequently for ticks and lice.

Anemia Prevention in Piglets

Pigs usually get all the iron and copper they need from rooting in the soil and eating green plants. However, for the 1st month after they're born, piglets are dependent on their mother's milk for the main part of their nutritional needs. Everything would be fine except that sow's milk doesn't contain enough iron or copper to supply the piglets' need for these minerals. Therefore, young pigs should receive an iron injection to prevent anemia and to build the blood they will need in order to grow.

The product you want to inject is ferric oxide (iron) stabilized with dextran. It comes under various names according to manufacturer; a few of them are Pig-Dex 100 (Cyanamid), Myofer 100 (Hoechst AG), and Ferro-Mycin 100 (Anchor Laboratories, Inc.). There is no difference between any of these products except price.

The dosage depends on the piglet's age. Each piglet 2–4 days old should receive 1 cm³ which equals 1 cc or 100 mg, depending on how the medicine is labeled. Piglets 1–6 weeks old should receive 2 cm³ equal to 2 cc or 200 mg. Piglets older than 6 weeks should already be weaned and receiving the iron and copper they need from dirt and green feed.

How to Inject Your Piglets

First, take your syringe apart and sterilize all the pieces and needles by boiling them in water for 10 minutes or longer. Reassemble the syringe, making sure it's dry and that no water remains inside. An easy way to do this is to lay several sheets of clean, unused toiletpaper on a flat surface. Then take the pieces of your syringe out of the pot you've boiled them in and lay them on the paper. Tap them gently on the paper and you'll remove most of the water. Blow out the drops that are left or wipe them out with unused toiletpaper or clean, sterile cotton. Don't forget to blow the water out of the needles.

Reassemble the syringe (making sure your hands have been well scrubbed with soap and water, then dried and swabbed with alcohol to disinfect them), and put on a sterilized needle. This needle will only be used to remove the iron solution from its bottle. Clean the rubber top of the bottle with alcohol, let it dry, and then, with the syringe, remove the amount of iron you need to inject (see Chapter 7, Syringes, p. 26).

Hold the syringe with the needle pointing straight up in the air in order not to spill any of the iron. Take off the needle you used to remove the solution and put on a sterilized number 20 needle. Still holding the syringe with the needle pointed up, carefully and slowly depress the plunger to expel any air that may be inside. Now you are ready to make the injection.

One major problem is how to hold the piglet so it doesn't squirm around and try to get free while you're injecting it. After fighting with my first five piglets I finally figured out an almost foolproof method of holding them. You, the person giving the injection, should sit on a bench or chair with your feet touching the ground and your knees spread apart. Since the injection will be made intramuscularly, in the middle of the thigh or ass muscle, another person suspends the piglet, holding onto one rear foot with each hand, so that its back faces you. Your helper lowers the piglet between your legs (don't pay any attention to its squealing) while you squeeze it between your knees so that it can't move. The other person should hold the piglet with its rear legs spread a normal distance apart. It's a two-person operation, so make sure your helper doesn't let go until the piglet is injected and ready to be sent back to its mother (see Figure 77).

Next clean the injection site with a piece of sterile cotton dipped in alcohol. Pull the skin to one side with your thumb and exert a little downward pressure with it. Hold the syringe perpendicular to the pig's skin and insert the needle slowly. A pig's skin is tough so you'll feel a little resistance at first, then the needle passes easily. Insert the needle one half of its length, or half an inch. Make sure you're using a number 20 needle!

At this point check to see if you've inserted the needle in a vein. Pull the plunger of the syringe out a little bit. If blood enters you'll be able to tell because it won't mix with the iron solution. If you are in a vein you've inserted the needle too far. Pull it out a little bit. Repeat the same operation to see if the needle is still in the vein; if it isn't, inject the iron slowly and steadily.

As you remove the needle make sure you take it out perpendicular to the pig's skin, the same way you inserted it. If you don't, you may rip the piglet's leg muscle creating a possible infection site and potentially causing the animal to go lame.

After removing the needle, release your thumb and let the piglet's skin return to its normal position. Clean the injection site with a piece of cotton dipped in alcohol. Take a close look to see if blood is oozing from the needle mark. If it is, apply pressure with your thumb and the bleeding should stop in a matter of seconds.

Let the piglet go. It will act dazed for a minute or two and may even stumble a bit as it walks, then it'll head directly for its sow. Most of the

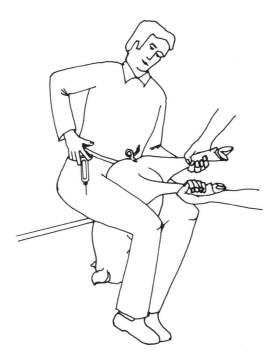

Figure 77.   How to hold a piglet while giving it an iron injection.

piglets I've injected against anemia have laid down to rest for about half an hour after getting their shot. This is a normal reaction for piglets.

Suggestions

1. Don't hurry! Take your time, the piglet isn't going anywhere.
2. Make sure the sow is placed in a pen out of sight of her piglets. If not, as you inject them and they squeal she may fight to get loose to protect them. And an angry sow is no one's idea of fun.
3. A good way to hold little pigs while they are waiting for their shot is inside a burlap or plastic grain bag. That way you know which has received its injection and which hasn't.
4. Giving an iron shot is a convenient time to check for ticks, fleas, and lice.

17

MINOR OPERATIONS

Castration

The main reason for castrating a male animal is to make it grow a more desirable quality of meat. When its testicles are removed or the blood supply to them is cut off, causing the testicles to die and eventually wither away, the production of male sex hormones ceases. Without these hormones the animal will put more of its growth into fat than it would have done otherwise.

Meat quality is determined by the amount of muscle tissue and fat it contains. A castrated male puts on weight more quickly and grows tissue with a higher percentage of fat than an uncastrated animal. Since fat content determines meat flavor a castrated animal will produce better quality meat.

Because castrated animals don't produce male sex hormones they have diminished sexual instincts and won't fight among themselves to prove superiority over other males. With fewer distractions their main interest is eating. They have a more docile temperment and are easier to handle when examining, transporting, injecting, vaccinating, or ridding of ticks, fleas, and lice. They are also easier to work with, as in the case of oxen.

Proper Conditions

The younger an animal is castrated the better; in most cases it certainly should be done before weaning. A young animal in good health receives a smaller shock to its system and recovers more quickly from the wound than does an older one. Any animal you castrate should be in good health and should not be too thin or have any kind of sickness. If it is in poor physical condition, underweight, or sick the animal's natural defenses will be weak. As a result, castration, which normally would have been a simple, minor operation may be a severe and dangerous one, leaving the animal in such a weakened condition that it is easily attacked by infection or disease, or even so debilitated that it may die.

It is best to castrate in dry weather and during a season when there are few or no flies. When it is wet or raining there is a greater chance of inflammation or infection setting in. The operation should be performed in clean areas, away from mud, sewage, garbage, manure, and dust, all of which are perfect media for various kinds of microorganisms, one of the most dangerous of which is tetanus. The best spot to castrate large animals, such as boars or rams, that need to be taken off their feet and tied so as not to struggle, is in clean grass or pasture. Small animals, such as piglets, fit well into your lap.

How to Castrate With a Knife

First, sharpen your knife blade. All animals with wool or hair growing on, around, or near their testicles should have it cut as close to the skin as possible with scissors. The scrotum and surrounding area of the groin should be washed thoroughly with soap, rinsed clean to remove any dirt and manure, and dried. Warm water is best for washing as it usually causes the animal to relax. Cold and hot water can shock and scald the animal, agitating it and causing it to struggle to get free. Drying is done easily with toiletpaper or paper towels.

Disinfect the scrotum and surrounding area of the groin with a piece of sterile cotton dipped in alcohol. Clean the area well and let it dry. The helper or helpers should hold the animal securely so that it can't move, to prevent it from getting dirty again.

The person doing the castration should wash his or her hands and arms up to the elbow, rinse them off, and dry them. First sharpen, and then disinfect the knife by dipping a piece of sterile cotton in alcohol or iodine and completely cleaning the sharpened blade.

Place the knife in a sterilized metal bowl or on a clean, unused piece of paper, either toiletpaper or a paper towel. From this point on no one but the castrator should touch the knife.

The animal is held on its back with all four legs tied together securely; the castrator kneels behind it. Take the scrotum in your left hand if you're a righty and in your right if you're left-handed. You will notice a line in the skin separating the two sides of the sac. Hold the scrotum so that your hand is between the animal's body and the right testicle. The testicle should now be above your hand. Squeezing hard, force the testicle to the side and tip of the scrotum. It should be to the right of the center line and pushed to the very end of the sack so that no loose skin remains and the shape of the testicle is clearly seen (see Figure 78).

Hold the knife firmly and make a straight incision in the middle of the skin covering the testicle. Begin a little bit above the testicle and end a little bit below it (see Figure 79). Maintain the pressure from below by squeezing upward with your other hand. You will notice that the underlying tissue is white; cut through this layer. If the incision was long enough the testicle will be forced out through the slit by squeezing (see Figure 80). Put the knife into its sterilized metal bowl or onto clean paper.

The testicle is surrounded by a very thin, clear to white-colored membrane which is attached to the inner wall of the scrotum. This should be stripped off with your fingers, at the same time pulling out moderately on the testicle itself and pushing the scrotum in the opposite direction. As the

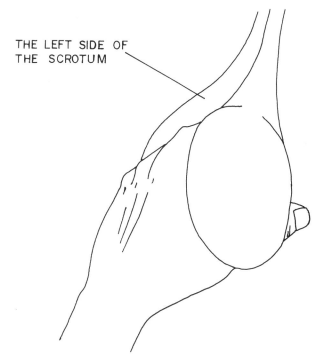

THE LEFT SIDE OF
THE SCROTUM

Figure 78.   The testicle is forced to the side and tip of the scrotum.

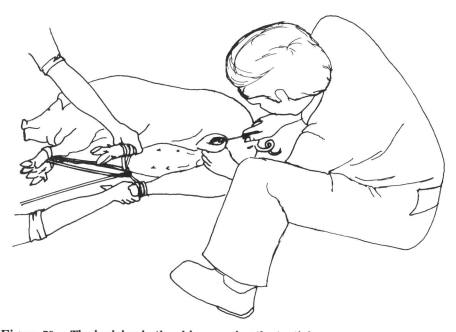

Figure 79.   The incision in the skin covering the testicle.

membrane is stripped off, the whitish cord, by which the testicle is suspended, and the purple artery, which brings blood to the testicle, will be exposed. Pull out on the testicle and push up on the scrotum in order to bring as much of the cord and artery through the knife incision as possible (see Figure 81).

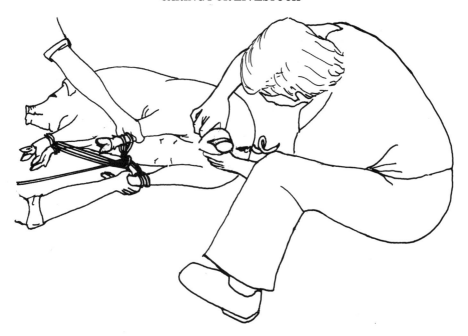

Figure 80.   Squeeze the testicle through the incision in the scrotum.

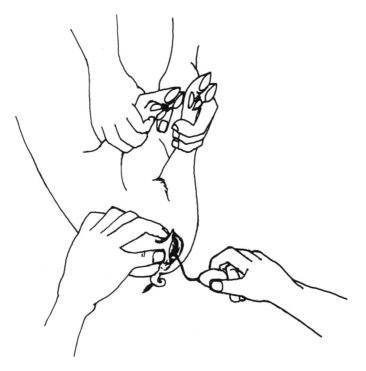

Figure 81.   Pull the testicle and the testicular cord and artery through the incision.

At this point there are two ways to cut off the blood supply to the testicle: sew a tight knot (see Figures 82a-e) around the testicular artery with a sterilized needle and disinfected suturing thread or heavy-duty cotton sewing thread (see Figure 83), or by pinching the artery between

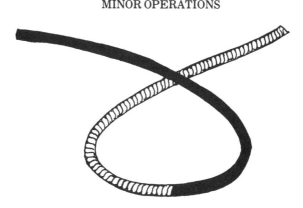

Figure 82a. Five steps to tying a surgeon's knot that will not slip. Step one.

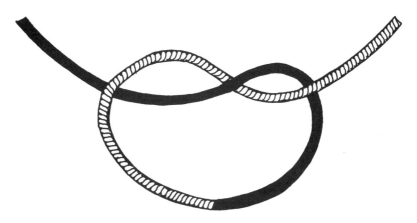

Figure 82b. Five steps to tying a surgeon's knot that will not slip. Step two.

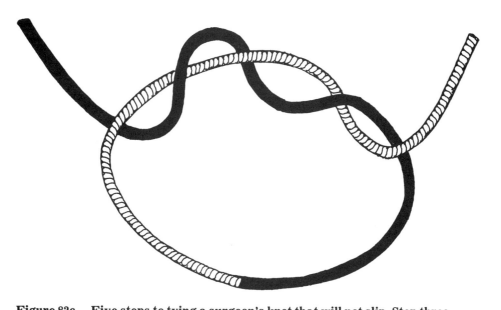

Figure 82c. Five steps to tying a surgeon's knot that will not slip. Step three.

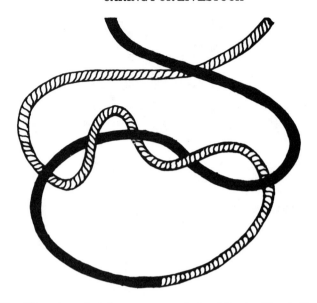

Figure 82d.   Five steps to tying a surgeon's knot that will not slip. Step four.

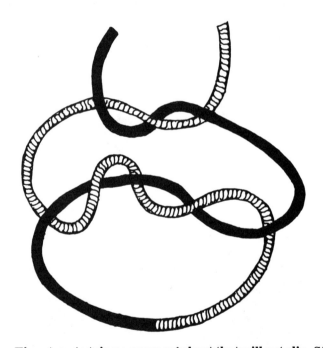

Figure 82e.   Five steps to tying a surgeon's knot that will not slip. Step five.

your fingers as hard as you can and turning the testicle in one direction until the artery snaps off below the pressure point. Both of these are acceptable techniques if caution is used. Make sure the knot is tied tightly and that the needle passes through the artery several times so the knot doesn't slip off (don't just wind the thread around the outside of the artery).

The following is a description of how to pinch the artery and turn it on itself. One of the helpers feels where the cord and artery pass through the

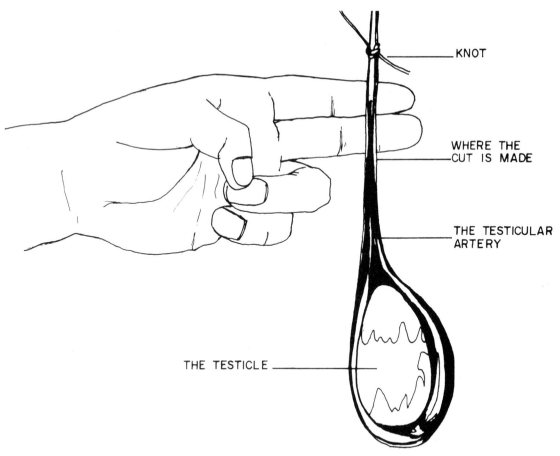

KNOT

WHERE THE
CUT IS MADE

THE TESTICULAR
ARTERY

THE TESTICLE

Figure 83.   Measure two finger widths below the knot to make your cut.

animal's body into the scrotum. You'll find that they feel like a hard, slippery rope. With his or her thumb and first finger, or with both hands if he or she is not strong enough to do it with one, the helper squeezes the cord and artery as hard and as close to the animal's body as possible (see Figure 84). This creates a tourniquet effect and cuts off the blood supply to the testicle.

Using both hands the castrator begins to turn the testicle in one direction or the other, but always in the same direction. At first it will be easy, but the testicle is slippery and as the cord and artery are turned again and again on themselves they tighten, making it more difficult. As the testicle is turned it should be pulled out from the body of the animal with a steady, moderate tension. After a minute or two of turning the castrator will feel a small snap. This is the cord beginning to break. In a few more seconds the cord breaks completely and one testicle has been removed.

The helper should keep squeezing the cord and artery as hard as possible for at least 15 seconds after the testicle has been removed. This steady pressure on the artery prevents serious bleeding.

The left testicle is removed in the same way: by making an incision, stripping off the membrane, pulling out through the slit as much of the cord and artery as possible, squeezing them as hard as you can close to the body and twisting the testicle. Remember to maintain pressure on the artery after the testicle is removed. With the other method, instead of

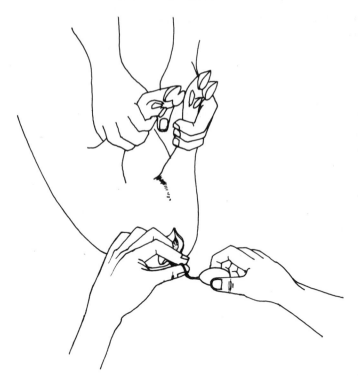

Figure 84.   Squeeze the testicular cord and artery as hard as you can close to the pig's body.

twisting the testicle to break the cord and artery they are tied with a knot and are then cut off two fingers width below the knot.

If the animal bleeds at all I like to use salt to stop it. Spread the cut apart and drop salt into the scrotum; it will cause the blood to coagulate. Finally, dip a piece of sterile cotton into an iodine disinfectant and paint both cuts, the scrotum and surrounding area of the groin to prevent infection.

Untie the animal's legs and get it to its feet. It should be kept in a clean area, preferably where there is grass, and in the shade out of the sun, to recover from the operation. The animal needs access to clean water at all times. It will be stiff and walk bowlegged for the first day but afterward will feel little or no pain. Within 2-3 days the wounds will close up and they will have healed almost completely in a week.

For a few days after being castrated the animal should not be agitated, made to walk long distances, carry heavy loads, or be worked. If so, it is liable to hemorrhage (lose a large amount of blood) and may bleed to death.

Piglets

Piglets are castrated when very young because they are easy to handle, heal quickly, and will begin to grow a tastier quality of meat faster than an uncastrated animal.

Unweaned piglets can be castrated at any time between birth and 4 weeks. I like to do it at 2 weeks when their testicles are the size of small marbles and easy to hold on to. At that point they will have had 14 days to get a good growing start and will have another 2 weeks to gain strength before being weaned at 1 month.

The procedure is the same for any other animal except that piglets are held on their backs and squeezed tightly between the castrator's legs. The castrator sits on a chair or bench with his or her feet touching the ground. The piglet is upside down with its head facing away from the castrator; there is no need to tie it. A helper stands in front of the piglet holding its left front and rear legs in his or her left hand and its right front and rear legs in his right hand (see Figure 85).

Uncastrated piglets should be held in a burlap or plastic grain bag while they wait their turn. The sow is always kept out of sight of the castration! If not, she may break loose and attack if she sees her young struggling and hears them squealing in fear and pain. As soon as each piglet is castrated turn it loose to find its way back to its mother. Usually, as soon as one reaches her she will lose interest in the others in order to comfort it.

Boars

Boars older than 6 weeks have to be restrained to be castrated. Tie the back legs together. Pass the free end of the rope around the front legs and tie them together. Then take the free end and loop it over the rope

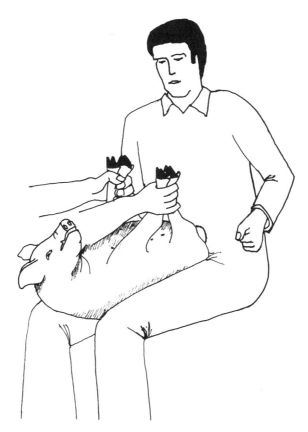

Figure 85.   How to hold a piglet to castrate it.

connecting the hind legs. Stand off to the side of the animal, and near its shoulders, with the end of the rope in your hands. Pull. This will bring the front and hind legs together knocking the animal off its feet. Now, roll the boar onto its back and tie the rope off (see Figures 86a–d).

Sometimes large boars just won't stop fighting against their bonds if held on their backs. If this happens roll the animal onto its side and castrate from that position. Whether it is on its back or side you will need several people to hold it still. One thing to remember is that quite often a boar can be kept from fighting as it is being tied if you scratch its back.

Rams and Bucks

Only a small percentage of rams will be saved for breeding, the rest should be castrated between their first and second week. At the same time all lambs, male and female, should be docked—have their tails cut

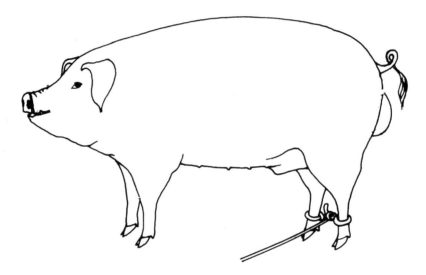

Figure 86a.   Tie the boar's hind legs.

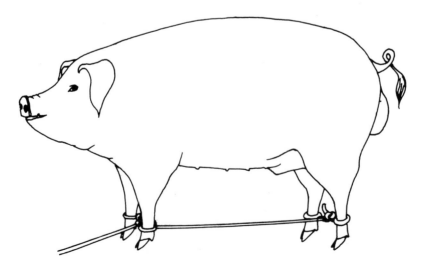

Figure 86b.   Tie the front legs together with the same rope.

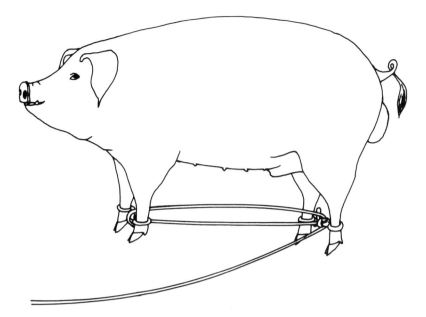

Figure 86c.   Pass the free end of the rope in between the tied-together hind legs.

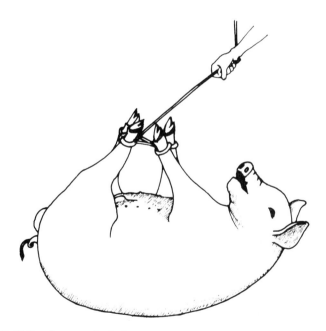

Figure 86d.   Pull the free end of the rope to draw the boar's legs together and take it off its feet. Then tie the rope securely.

off, leaving about a 1-inch stub (see "Docking," p. 221).

Rams of any age are the easiest animals to castrate. They don't need to be tied and can be held on their backs by one person. Goat bucks are castrated just like rams. A young buck can be held still by hand, while an older one should be tied. Look out for the hooves, they pack a powerful wallop.

Bulls

The younger a bull calf is when castrated the easier it is to control and the quicker it recovers. It is possible to do the castration 2-3 days after birth, holding it immobile on its back or tying it if necessary.

At 2 months or older the calf should be castrated while standing. A halter is put over the head and snugged off to a post. The helper pushes the animal's hindquarters up against a fence while holding its tail firmly at the base. If the calf struggles or kicks it is easily controlled by forcing up hard on the base of the tail and pushing it above the back. This puts strong pressure on the nerves located there and usually changes the calf's mind about kicking (see Figure 87). The castrator stands behind the animal's legs and operates with the usual technique.

Mature bulls are big, strong, unpredictable when enraged, and are not worth arguing with. Restrain them well! One method is to tie their halter to a post and wedge them against a fence as with bull calves. They are subdued not only by means of the tail but also by a rope tied around the crop and then the flank. Snugged down tightly this rope will keep the animal from kicking (see Figure 88). If this doesn't keep it still take it off its feet and immobilize it (see Figure 89).

If the bull is to be castrated for use as an ox wait until it is at least 6 months old. By that time the desirable masculine physical characteristics for its future use, such as muscling, broadened shoulders, and thickened head will have developed.

Castration Without Surgery

Two other methods of castration, elastration and the use of an emasculatome, are in wide use. Both work by cutting off the blood supply to the testicles, which causes them to die and wither away. With elastration this occurs within several weeks; when using an emasculatome it happens in 4-6 weeks.

Both are easier to perform than surgical castrations but cost more as special tools are needed. I don't believe the cost of the tools necessary for either type of bloodless castration is justified unless you have many animals or just can't stand the sight of blood. I'm still prejudiced in favor of my battered and inexpensive electrician's knife. However, the great advantage of both methods is that they can be used all year long. They are both bloodless, since there is no incision, and therefore pose no danger of fly-borne infection. Of the two, the emasculatome is preferable because there is no pain and no possibility of mistake.

Elastration

In elastration, an instrument is used to stretch a small and thick rubber band. The band is put around the scrotum close to the animal's groin. The pressure the band exerts cuts off the blood supply to the testicles and the scrotum. In a few weeks they die, dry up, and fall off.

The bands cause swelling and pain for a few days, and do break from time to time. Since one break of a band is all you need for failure, I don't recommend this method.

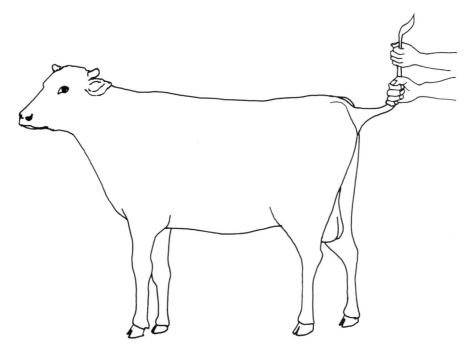

Figure 87.   Force up hard on the base of the tail to keep a bull calf from kicking.

Using an Emasculatome

The emasculatome, also known as Burdizzo Pincers, looks like bolt cutters. It works by crushing both the testicular cord and artery when its jaws are closed on them. The jaws don't quite fit together and won't damage the scrotum itself. The emasculatome works best on animals with hanging scrotums such as bulls, horses, and sheep, and not as easily on those with scrotums held close to the body, such as pigs (see Figure 90).

The pincers are slipped over a side of the scrotum 1-½ to 2″ above the testicle. (The distance above the testicle is not too critical.) Push the testicular cord to the outside of the scrotum as far as it will go; close the jaws and squeeze for at least 5 seconds, which is the time needed to completely crush the cord. Do the same on the other side (see Figure 91).

Docking

Lambs should have their tails docked (cut short) when they are 1-2 weeks old. At that age, and up to a month, it is an easy operation from which the young animals recover very quickly. Since castrations of young rams that won't be used for breeding are done at the same age, you can dock and castrate them on the same day.

The tail is docked for health reasons and to facilitate the breeding of ewes when they become sexually mature. Also, the long tail of a mature sheep is often wet with feces and provides a perfect environment in which flies can lay their eggs and for the development of larvae and maggots.

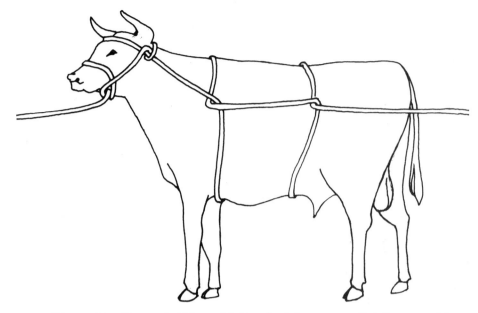

Figure 88.   Keep a bull from kicking by tying a rope tightly around its crop and flank.

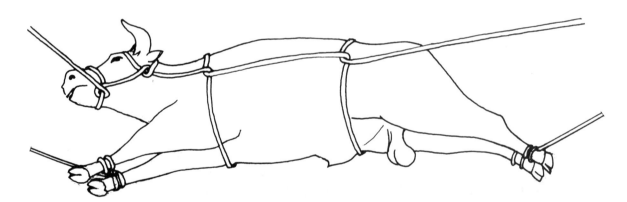

Figure 89.   Take the bull off its feet to subdue it.

The lamb is held immobile by a helper while you put an emascula-tome (the Small Size Burdizzo Castrator Cord-Stop is the best one made) over its tail, and cut it off an inch from the animal's anus. Immediately apply iodine to the little bit of tail that remains. Then give the lamb an intramuscular injection of tetanus antitoxin to give it passive immunity to tetanus in case an infection develops in its tail stump before it heals. Turn lambs out onto the clean pasture with their ewes after the operation. It is surprising how quickly they return to nursing and forget about the tail.

Docking with an emasculatome is a very safe procedure because it crushes the blood vessels in the tail stub and prevents the possibility of hemorrhage.

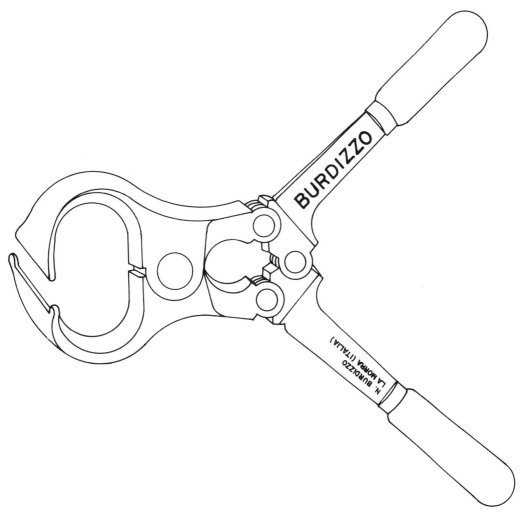

Figure 90. The burdizzo emasculatome.

Dehorning

The removal of the horns of your cattle and goats is a common and uncomplicated operation that is done with everyone's safety and well-being in mind. The best time to do the operation is when animals are still quite young, as calves or kids, but adults can also have their "hat racks" removed, though it is usually a job for your veterinarian.

Calves

Calves are disbudded when only a few days old and are easily manageable. There are two recommended disbudding techniques—gouging and the electric iron. There are two which often cause problems—caustic ointment and the elastrator.

The gouger is a tool with a sharp-bladed cutting head that fits over the calf's horn bud. It has two long wooden handles that remain close together when the cutting head is open. In order to cut out the bud the handles are pulled apart rapidly as downward pressure is exerted. This

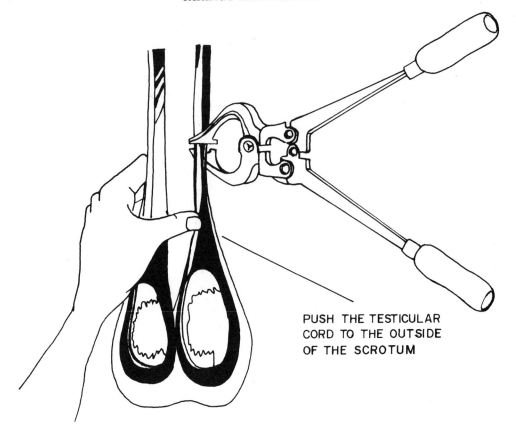

PUSH THE TESTICULAR
CORD TO THE OUTSIDE
OF THE SCROTUM

Figure 91.   How to use the emasculatome.

scoops the horn bud out at its root leaving a cleanly cut depression in the head.

Use a dehorning powder after removing both buds. Sprinkle it freely on the wounds to stop the bleeding; it will cause the blood to coagulate in a few minutes. In case the bleeding doesn't stop put cotton bandages over each hole and wrap more of the material around the calf's head. Tie it off tightly with enough pressure to stop the blood flow. Your little calf should look like a concussion victim or a mummy with all the cotton bandage it will be wearing. This indignity lasts only a day and then the bandage is removed. Paint the wounds, skin, and hair around them with an antiseptic and a good fly repellent since the open holes are a choice spot for flies to lay their eggs.

The other recommended dehorning method is with an electric dehorning iron, a tool that looks like a soldering iron. The calf is restrained by a helper and held immobile while you snip off the hair around its horn buds with scissors. Then the iron is heated until it is red-hot and will scorch wood; try it on a piece of pine if you are not sure if it is hot enough. Place the tip of the iron on the bud and rotate it around the bud base.

In spite of the calf's blood-curdling bawling and the stench of burning horn, keep the iron on the bud for at least 6 seconds. Even though it doesn't feel like those 6 seconds will ever end, it is very important to burn out all of the bud tissue so that a misshapen horn doesn't develop. Most disbudding problems are caused by not applying the iron long enough, rather than too much.

After finishing the first bud let the iron reheat and do the second one.

Disinfect the holes with iodine and apply a fly repellent. The calf is none the worse for wear and immediately forgets the loss of its buds if allowed to suckle its mother, or if given a bottle of warm milk.

The buds may also be removed by using a caustic ointment, but I think this is dangerous and I wouldn't use it on my animals. The hair is clipped around the buds as described above. Petroleum jelly is put on in a good coating around the eyes and in a circle around the base of the buds. The base of the buds and the buds themselves are left ungreased. Now the caustic ointment is painted onto the base of the buds and covers the buds as well. The ointment kills the horn tissue and no horns will grow.

But the major danger is that caustic ointments burn any live tissue they come in contact with. They run when they get wet, either from the rain or a watering trough, and can blind or seriously injure the treated calf or the other calves it frolics with. As the calf suckles its dam it commonly butts her in the udder to hasten the letdown of her milk. If it has a caustic ointment on its head it can burn her udder. Therefore, steer clear of this disbudding method—it is too much trouble and can be dangerous.

The other treatment to avoid is the use of an elastrator. This tool puts a thick, little rubber band around the very bottom of the base of the bud after you have cut off the hair there. The pressure exerted by the squeezing rubber band cuts off the blood supply to the horn tissue and it dies. Eventually the horn falls off, but only if the rubber band doesn't break. If it wasn't put on right to begin with the horn keeps growing and you've got to dehorn it again. Finally, it hurts the calf and may cause it to go off feed or even injure itself as it rubs its horns against a pen wall or the ground to stop the pain.

Mature Cattle

Dehorning adult cattle is a job for your veterinarian. The cow is held immobile in a squeeze chute or by some other means while the horns are cut off. No matter how you restrain the animal it must not be able to move its head at all during the operation.

The cutting jaws of a long-handled dehorner (see Figure 92) are placed around the base of the horn as close to the head as possible in cows and young bulls with small to medium-sized horns. As the handles are pulled together the jaws close, cutting off the horn. Generally a stream of blood shoots out of an artery lying close to the surface of the head. Your veterinarian will slow the bleeding by cauterizing the artery or by crushing it with a forceps, and then will dust on a powder which will cause the blood to coagulate.

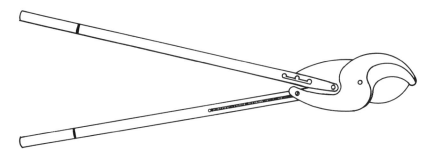

Figure 92. A cattle dehorner.

Animals with horns that are thick at the base (mature bulls and older cows) are dehorned with a special electric saw or a handsaw. If a manual dehorner were used the horn could crack and split externally, or even inside the animal's head, and the skull itself could fracture. When sawing the horns off by hand the cow or bull is injected intramuscularly close to the base of each horn with a local anesthetic to deaden the nerves there. If this isn't done and you begin sawing away you will get an immediate test of how well you restrained the animal to begin with. Don't underestimate how sensitive the area around the base of the horns is. I once saw an enraged Brahma cow, that had been securely tied up and "restrained" destroy a corral sorting pen because its owner didn't see the need to give it an anesthetic before attempting to cut its horns off with a handsaw. That was a cost-saving measure he has never repeated again.

Kids

Kids are dehorned in much the same way calves are. They are restrained by an assistant so they can't move (a good way is to squeeze its body between your knees and hold its head with your hands) and the hair around the base of the horn buds is snipped off with scissors. The electric iron, heated a deep red, is placed on the center of the bud and rotated around while pressing down for 6 seconds. This will flatten the bud to the head, leaving a tiny circle of horn tissue around the center you have burned out. Even off this outer portion with the iron until it, too, is flush with the head. Repeat the operation on the second bud, apply Gentian Violet, and paint on a fly repellent.

Kids should be disbudded on their 4th day. This gives them a few days to gain strength after birth and doesn't cause a setback to their growth as debudding at a later age might. Before proceeding, determine whether your kids are horned or hornless. This may sound foolish but you would be surprised how many people don't know when disbudding time comes. Kids that are polled, naturally hornless, have heads that are somewhat rounded and the hair covering the spots the buds should occupy is straight. Horned kids have flatter heads and a little curl directly above each bud.

When they are 3 days old snip off all the hair around the buds. If kids are going to be raised on a bottle take their mothers from them. Turn the nannies out with the herd and disinfect their kidding pens thoroughly so they can't smell their kids when they return. The bedding should be changed and they should have their feeding racks filled with enticing, fresh-cut green grass to occupy them and keep them from fretting about their missing young. Kids should be used to nursing from a bottle before they are disbudded so that giving them a bottle after the operation works to settle them down and make them forget the recent pain. Kids that will be left on their mothers milk should be allowed to nurse them and huddle in their warmth and comfort after disbudding.

The bud scabs fall off in a few days but the kid's head will be sore for a week or two. Don't be surprised if it bawls in pain if it bangs it during these 2 weeks.

Mature Goats

Once again, this is a job for your verterinarian unless you have a lot of animals and can learn to dehorn them yourself. If you decide to do your own dehorning call the vet out to teach you how to do it, and have him or her stand right by you as you do your first couple of animals.

Restrain the animal well and make sure it can't move its head. Give it intramuscular injections of a local anesthetic and a tranquilizer into the flesh of the head close to the base of its horn. Then cut the horn and a strip of skin as close to the head as you can with a medium-toothed hacksaw. You should actually cut off a swath of hair and skin at the base of the horn; the hacksaw is held flush to the head and the cut conforms to the head contour. If done correctly you will see a big, bloody hole where there was once a horn.

The arteries in the base of the horn should be exposed when it is cut off. These are stripped out or cauterized with a hot iron to stop the bleeding. Follow your veterinarian's instructions carefully on this. If the dehorned goat doesn't stop bleeding, pour on a coagulant powder and put a couple of swatches of sterile cotton gauze on top of each hole and then wrap a cotton bandage over them and around its head. The bandage pressure will stop the bleeding before too long; after a day it is taken off.

After cutting off the first horn do the second one in the same way. Disinfect the holes and paint on a fly repellent around the whole area.

Removal of Extra Teats in Dairy Cattle

Extra, nonfunctional teats are sometimes found on heifers' udders. It is a good idea to remove them from dairy heifers in order to reduce irritation, facilitate milking, and to prevent possible outbreaks of mastitis.

The operation is a simple one that is done when heifers are 3–8 months old and their udders are large enough to work on. The animal is restrained well so it can't move or kick and the extra teats are cut flush to the udder with sharp, sterilized scissors. The wound is disinfected with an antiseptic and a fly repellent is painted on.

Removing the Musk Glands of Male Goats

As the comedian Jimmy Durante said so eloquently, "the nose knows." That is the literal truth about male goats. They love to leave a smelly autograph on whatever they consider to be theirs: you, their feeder, the females they breed, and the pens they occupy. Females also have musk glands, but they rarely become active.

Getting rid of these scent glands is easily done when kids are disbudded, since they are located right behind the buds (see Figure 93). If male kids are going to be castrated don't bother de-scenting them since the musk is only produced when male sex hormones are secreted. Without testicles the little buck won't produce the necessary hormones, and hence there will be no smell.

Kids' musk glands are darker than the surrounding skin and are easily seen if the hair behind the bud, in horned animals, or where the bud would be in hornless animals, is clipped away in an arc at least an inch wide. Adult males have the hair removed in the same area which exposes

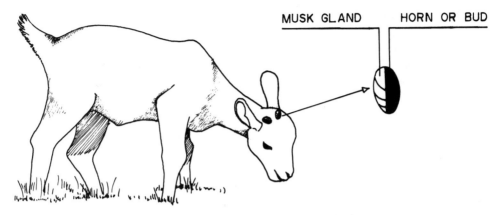

Figure 93.   The musk glands are located right behind the horns.

a thicker and shinier bit of skin than that adjoining it. If it is breeding season the glands will appear raised above the surface of the surrounding skin and will be wrinkled, with three folds on each side of them.

The glands are removed with the same electric iron which you use to dehorn. Heat it red-hot and burn the glands until they look like bone. Make sure you get all of it since part of the gland is under the base of the back part of the horn (or where it was before you removed it). The kid gets an intramuscular injection of tetanus antitoxin with a broad spectrum antibiotic to protect it against infections. Disinfect the wounds with an antiseptic and paint on fly repellent.

If the adult buck is hornless you can also use an electric iron on it. If it is horned, have your veterinarian remove its glands surgically at the same time its horns come off.

Abscesses

An abscess is a pus-filled spot in an animal's body that may be swollen and inflamed. It is usually caused by a bacterial infection. Most farm animals get abscesses from time to time and they usually go away of their own accord. It is best to not be in a rush to lance an abscess—cut it open with a surgical knife—until it is apparent it isn't going to break, drain, and heal internally.

Since abscesses are caused by many kinds of bacteria, including *Cornebacterium pyogenes, Bacteroides, E. coli, steptococci,* and *staphylococci* to name a few, it is a good idea for you or your veterinarian to remove a little bit of the abscess pus with a syringe and send it to a laboratory for culture. Ask the lab to determine what the infectious bacteria is and what drug it is sensitive to. In this way you'll be sure to use the correct drug for the specific microorganism. This will result in quicker cure and will avoid building up resistance to some other, incorrectly, used antibiotic.

Abscesses occur both internally and externally. Those that develop inside an animal, in its organs and tissues, should be handled by your veterinarian since neither diagnosis nor treatment is easy. Likewise, leave abscesses of the udder and the throat and neck to the professional because they are too dangerous to afford to make a mistake on. However, any abscess that appears on the surface of the animal's body, on any part except the udder, neck, or throat, you can treat yourself.

First determine that the swollen abscess does in fact contain pus, and not blood, by removing some of its fluid with a syringe with a sterilized needle. If the swelling contains blood that has seeped into it from the surrounding tissue the animal could bleed to death when you lance what you think is an ordinary pus-filled abscess. All of a sudden a very routine and minor surgery can become a life and death situation. Don't learn the hard way!

Subdue the animal securely and keep it in a sick pen or some other area removed from its pen or herdmates. If the animal has long hair, trim it off around the abscess and then wash the whole area with disinfectant. Lay a rag or feed bag on the ground underneath the abscess to collect its pus. Next put on a pair of sterile or disinfected rubber gloves and go to work on the abscess, which is usually the size of your fist, by opening it with a sterilized knife (see Figure 94a).

Make a vertical cut of at least 2 inches in a straight line toward the bottom of the swelling cutting from top to bottom (see Figure 94b). The cut is made at the bottom of the abscess so that all the pus can be squeezed out, allowing the wound to drain properly. If the cut were made higher up a pool of pus might collect in the bottom of the abscess, and, no matter how well you cleaned it out, drainage would be poor, healing would be delayed, and reinfection could occur.

After making the incision widen the slit by removing a little bit of skin parallel to the cut with the same knife (wash it in disinfectant before doing this) or with a sterilized pair of scissors (see Figures 94c and d). What we are trying to do is create a wide enough opening so that the cut won't close up on itself and thereby give any infectious bacteria left inside the chance to start the whole disease process over again. With a wide slit drainage will be good and the inside of the abscess will heal quickly.

Disinfect your hands and squeeze the pus out of the abscess working from the top to the bottom and from the surrounding area into the center. (see Figure 94e). The pus that flows out may be as thin as milk or as thick as processed cheese; it is usually creamy, yellow, or green in color. As this pus, which contains huge numbers of the infective bacteria, is squeezed out it falls onto the rag or feedbag you have placed on the ground to absorb it. Keep squeezing until you can't get any more out.

The now deflated abscess should be rinsed out with a noncaustic disinfectant (one that won't burn the tissue). Make sure you have cleaned all of it and that no pus remains inside. You may have to repeat the rinsing a couple of times to be sure you have reached all of the interior surface. Dry the cut and exterior with a clean paper towel. At this point it is a good idea to double-check yourself by opening the cut and spraying an aerosol antiseptic into the wound and around the outside of the opening as well. A broad spectrum antibiotic in a liquid solution may be sprayed into the empty abscess or an intramuscular injection may be given. I like the latter because of its systemic action.

Before releasing the animal have a helper remove the pus-filled rag or feedbag. It is carried to a safe place without allowing it to drip; there it is doused with gasoline and set on fire. This prevents other animals from coming in contact with the infectious bacteria. The floor where the operation took place is disinfected, as are your gloves, the knife, and your

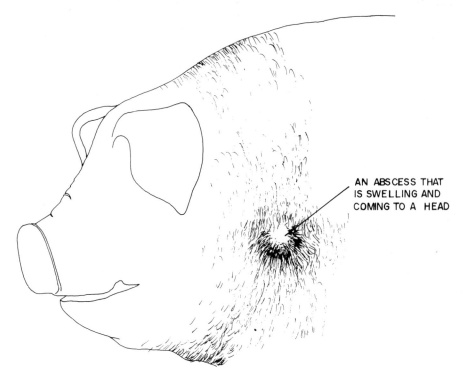

AN ABSCESS THAT
IS SWELLING AND
COMING TO A HEAD

Figure 94a.   Trim the hair around an abscess and disinfect it.

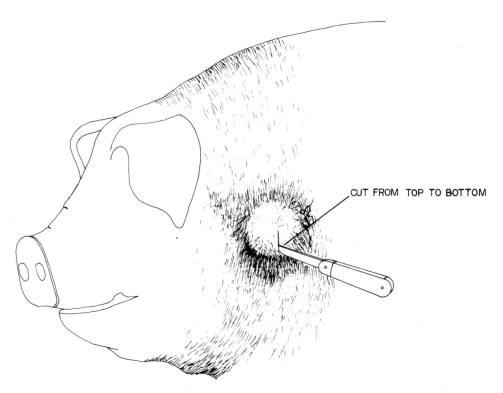

CUT FROM TOP TO BOTTOM

Figure 94b.   Make a 2-inch incision towards the bottom of the abscess.

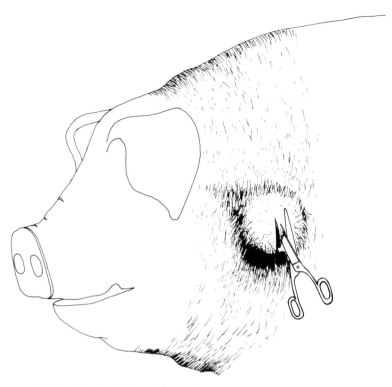

Figure 94c.   Widen the incision with a scissors so that it drains properly.

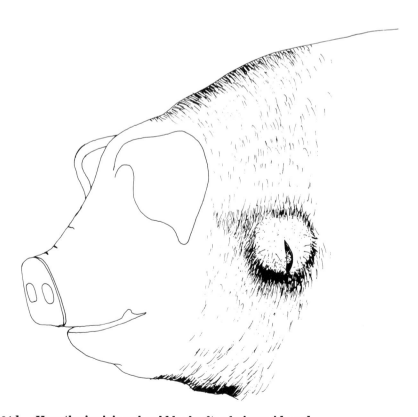

Figure 94d.   How the incision should look after being widened.

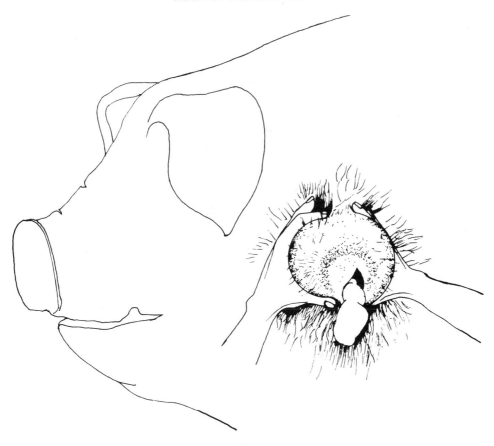

Figure 94e.   Squeeze all the pus out of the abscess.

hands. The treated animal is held in a disinfected sick pen or corral and
separated from its herdmates for several days to a week to give the
wound time to drain and heal. Inspect the wound daily and maintain
treatment with the specific antibiotic called for. If flies are a problem
paint on a fly repellent.

Clipping of Eyeteeth in Piglets

Eyeteeth, also called *needleteeth*, are easily clipped at birth with a
pair of sterilized wire snippers or cutting pliers. (see Figure 95). The tips
of both the top and bottom eyeteeth are snipped off to prevent injury to
the sow's nipples and to the faces of littermates as they fight amongst
themselves. Only the tips of the eyeteeth are removed. If they are cut
closer to the gums the teeth can shatter, the gums may become infected
and the tongue may be cut as the piglet nurses.

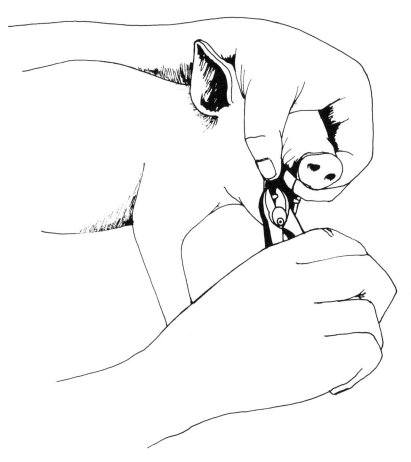

Figure 95. **Clip piglets' eyeteeth.**

18

REPRODUCTION

Puberty

Puberty, the age at which male and female animals reach sexual maturity and are able to reproduce, varies genetically among and within species. Goats reach puberty in half the time that it takes cattle to do so. In general, the smaller beef breeds become sexually mature faster than the larger ones.

The onset of puberty is also influenced by how well balanced an animal's diet is, whether its nutritional requirements are being met, its weight, the day length, the type and size of confinement system, and the number and sex of penmates. All over the world females of many species become sexually mature faster than males do: 2-4 months earlier in horses and cattle, and a few weeks in sheep, goats and pigs. If twins are separated at an early age and one is raised in a temperate zone and the other in the tropics, the tropical twin reaches puberty first.

Puberty, by definition, implies that animals are able to reproduce, but this does not necessarily mean that they will do so if bred at this age. Although males are physically capable at puberty of producing sperm that will fertilize female ova (eggs), the amount and quality of their sperm continues to increase for at least a year after attaining sexual maturity.

For the average age and range in age at puberty among the common farm animals consult the "Puberty Guide" on p. 235.

What Is Heat?

Once female animals reach puberty they develop a cyclical reproductive pattern known as the *estrous cycle*. At the point during the cycle when the female is sexually receptive to the male and will allow copulation to take place she is said to be in *heat*, or *estrus*. This period is

PUBERTY GUIDE

Animal Specie	Average Age At Puberty (in months)	Age Range At Puberty (in months)
Cattle (European breeds and crosses)	12	4–18
Cattle (Zebu types)		16–24
Horses	12–15	10–24
Sheep	9	5–12
Goats	5	4–8
Pigs	5–6	4–9
Rabbits	5–9	4–12

usually very short—a matter of hours to a few days—and must be watched for to calculate the best time for breeding to ensure fertilization and conception.

Each female within a species ovulates at some common point during or after the heat (with minor variations due to genetic differences) whether she has been bred or not. She passes one or more eggs from the ovaries, her chief reproductive organs, into tubes called the *oviducts* or *Fallopian tubes* which lead to the uterus. It is here in the upper part of the oviducts that fertilization of the female egg by the male reproductive cell, the sperm, must take place if offspring are to be produced.

The sperm race against time and incredible odds to reach the egg(s) before they lose strength and die. They swim through the female's vagina, where they are deposited by the male into the cervix when he ejaculates. The cervix is a short and very powerful muscular neck or ring connecting the vagina to the uterus. It is sealed, except during estrus and birth, with mucus to protect against contamination and infection. Passing through the cervix the sperm move into the bottom part of the uterus and along the curve of the two uterine horns until they reach the oviducts. As they swim through the oviducts one sperm must reach and penetrate each egg for their fertilization to occur.

If the egg and sperm unite they form a new cell that continues to move down the oviduct until it reaches the uterus. This new cell, the embryo, is nourished in the uterus, floating freely in the organ's secretions for 2–8 weeks, depending on the species, before gradually attaching to the inner wall. The embryo, now called a *fetus* and considered a young animal which has yet to be born, since cell differentiation has begun, develops, and grows very quickly.

If breeding doesn't occur, or if it takes place at the wrong time in the cycle, fertilization of the egg by a sperm will not be possible and the egg will die. If the female belongs to a species such as cattle or pigs, that is polyestrous (having more than one estrous cycle in a year), this process will repeat itself and the female will come back into heat in a number of weeks. If she is monoestrous (having only one estrous cycle each year), like dogs and foxes, she won't repeat the process until the same season next year. Monoestrous animals are also called seasonal breeders because they always come into heat at the same time each year unless under great stress.

How to Tell When Your Animals Are in Heat

Cows

Six to 10 hours before a "standing heat," the 18-hour period when a cow will let a bull mount her, the cow's vulva (the external part of her reproductive system that looks like lips) will swell a little bit, lubricate, and turn red. She walks around nosing, smelling, and sniffing other cows and mounts them, riding them for a few seconds as if she were a bull.

Following this preheat behavior the cow goes off feed and its milk production drops. The vulva is still wet and red and has swollen more than before. A clear mucus, stringlike in shape, is discharged from the vulva and is seen hanging down from it or else glued to the rump or tail. The cow is nervous and easily excited. She both rides other cows and stands immobile to be ridden herself. The pupils of her eyes dilate and she moos, bawls, and make enough racket so that her condition is unmistakable even if all of the other signs were missed.

Heat is more noticeable in heifers than in mature cows, some of whom show few really obvious symptoms other than a swollen, reddish vulva; and it is easier to spot in warm weather than in cold. You will know a "standing heat" has ended when the cow will no longer stand motionless waiting to be mounted when you exert downward pressure on her back or when a bull or other cow tries to ride her. However, up to 6 hours after the end of a "standing heat" is an excellent time to breed your animal in spite of what her body language is telling you (see "The Estrous Cycle Guide," p. 238).

Mares

Mares have the most variable heat period of all domestic farm animals: most show very obvious signs, some need to be "teased" by a stallion held on the other side of a wooden fence or with his head, but only his head, stuck through her stall door to bring on estrus, and another few commonly have silent heats in which no outward signs of estrus are noticed even though a stallion will detect it. Occasionally, mares will have split estrus during which they appear to be in heat for a few days and will let the stallion mount them. They then refuse to breed for a short period and finally, once again are receptive.

Mares in heat are very excitable, whinny a lot, and bother both mares and stallions by teasing them. In the presence of a stallion they squat and urinate frequently, often straining for some time after they have finished. The vulva is swollen, wet, and pinkish. Early in the heat a thick mucus discharge flows from and is spat out by the lips of the vulva as they expand and contract when the mare raises the base of her tail when being teased. The discharge increases in volume and becomes more watery as the mare gets closer and closer to ovulation (see Ovulation in "The Estrous Cycle Guide"). After ovulation, as heat dies down, this secretion flowing from the vulva decreases and becomes thicker again.

During the "standing heat" the mare and stallion's behaviors are violent. She bites and kicks at him as he moves close and tries to mount; he bites back, often savagely.

Sometimes mares, especially those with a foal, don't respond at all to teasing with a stallion when he is there, but do react once he is gone. For this reason it is important to keep good records of the animal's response to teasing in order to both determine if it is in heat and to hasten its onset.

Ewes

Ewes don't show the marked and obvious outward signs of heat that other species do although there is some variation by breed. Merinos are the most nervous and unsettled during estrus, and their vulvas become more visibly swollen and reddish than other sheep.

In general, all breeds' vulvas swell, turn red, and show a slight, thick mucus flow—enough to be noticed at the beginning of the heat if you look carefully. Soon afterward the mucus flows become heavier and clearer. Rams recognize the approach of estrus and search out ewes by smell for 2 days before they come into heat. By the rams' attempted mountings and teasings you should be able to identify estrous ewes.

Goat Does

Before coming into heat a milking goat's production increases, then falls for 1 or 2 days, and then increases again. Watch for this with your animals and see if you notice a pattern in milk production which will help you predict the beginning of estrus, especially in the good milkers.

As heat comes on the doe's vulva swells, turns red, and discharges a thick, stringy mucus flow which often collects on the tail or rump. She twitches her tail from side to side, bleats more than normally—sometimes so much you think she's in pain—and runs around in a nervous and excited way.

If there is a buck in with her he will mark her out for close personal attention by nipping and pawing and making "love talk" (which translates to me as deep, hoarse grunts). The doe squats, urinates and strains, and wags her tail, bleating in delight as he mounts her. Your normally demure and coy doe is an enthusiastic breeder. If she is running with other does and you don't have a buck she will mount and be mounted by her penmates. If you have neither buck nor does your female in a "standing heat" will usually shake her tail, bleat approvingly, and assume the recognizable breeding position when petted on the back.

Sows

As the sow comes into heat she becomes restless, her feed consumption drops, and she mounts other females. She squats and urinates a lot, her vulva is swollen bright red, and it discharges a stringy mucus. Either the urine or the mucus contain sex-stimulating chemicals which attract the boar.

When the boar has been turned in with the sow he initiates his breeding courtship (discussed in "Male Breeding Behavior," p. 254). They

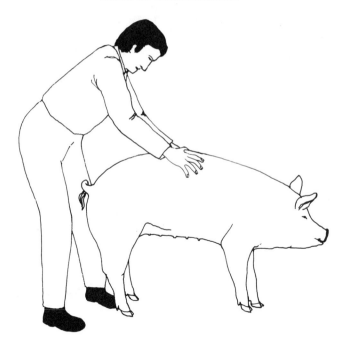

Figure 96.   Check if sows and gilts are in heat by pressing down on their backs.

grunt and talk to each other and the sow waits motionlessly and patiently in the hump-backed position of a "standing heat" for the male to mount her (see Figure 96).

Gilts typically develop swollen and red vulvas before other indications of estrus. They are more aggressive, or perhaps spirited, than sows, and will tease and then playfully resist and fight the boar before waiting immobile for the mount. Gilts often mount, nuzzle, and poke other gilts and sows with their snouts. Sows are gentler and calmer.

If you don't keep a boar some signs of heat may not be seen but you can count on a swelling and reddening of the vulva and the characteristic stance of the "standing heat."

Rabbit Does

Heat in rabbit does is a bit of a mystery as it is not clear yet whether they have true estrous cycles. However, nervousness, grunting sounds, the thumping of their feet on the floor of their cage, and rubbing their chins on any surface they can find are reliable indications that they are in heat. The combination of several of these signs should leave no doubt as to their condition.

The Estrous Cycle Guide

In the following guide you will be able to determine by species the normal range of the estrous cycle in days, its average length, how long heat lasts, when the best time to breed your female animals is, and when ovulation takes place.

Species	Average Length of Estrous Cycle (days)	Normal Range of Estrous Cycle (days)	How Long Heat Lasts	Best Time to Breed	Ovulation
Cow	21	18–24	1. Averages 18 hours 2. Ranges from 10–26 hours	From middle heat (9 hours) to 6 hours after it's over	10–12 hours after heat is over
Mare	21	19–26	1. Averages 6 days 2. Ranges from 2–10 days	1. In the last few days of heat 2. Breed twice 2 days apart	1–2 days before heat is over
Ewe	16½	14–20	1. Averages 30 hours 2. Ranges from 20–42 hours	Any time during heat	1. Toward the end of heat 2. Averages 24–30 hours after heat begins
Goat doe	19–20	18–21	1. Averages 48 hours 2. Ranges from 1–3½ days	Breed twice— once a day 2 days in a row	Toward the end of heat
Sow	21	18–24	1. Averages 40–70 hours 2. Ranges from 1–5 days	Breed the 1st and 2nd days of heat	46 hours after heat begins
Rabbit doe	Doesn't cycle regularly		Can last up to 30 days	As soon as heat is noticed	10½ hours after mating

The normal range of the estrous cycle is of value in highlighting the variability that exists within each species and is a reassuring guide (within limits) if you find that your animals aren't cycling in the same amount of time as their herdmates. The average cycle length is a quick estimate of when your animals should be cycling. Use both of these figures to determine the next heat and whether females have become pregnant after having been bred. For example, if your cow was bred 20 days ago and she doesn't come into heat in the next 4 days, chances are good that she is pregnant.

How long heat lasts can be of help in scheduling your breedings. The information on the best time to breed enables you to take best advantage of the animal's reproductive rhythm to have her impregnated. When ovulation takes place is of interest because it is the last major event of the estrous cycle and everything that leads up to it—the calculation of the number of days until the beginning of heat, how long heat will last, the selection of the male, the timing of the breeding, and so forth—is dependent on it for successful fertilization and pregnancy.

How to Select for and Induce
Early Puberty in Gilts

If gilts become sexually mature (reach puberty) earlier than the average for all female pigs, even if only by a few days, reproductive efficiency is increased. This means that the same number (all other factors that influence reproduction remaining unchanged) of piglets can be produced more quickly with less cost in feed, electricity, drugs, labor, and housing. This is, of course, one of the goals livestock breeders aim for: earlier reproductive capability in their breeding herds with no ill-effect on viability of the young or health of the dam.

It is possible to select for early puberty when designing your breeding program. Landrace gilts, of all the breeds that experiments have been held with so far, reach puberty earliest. However, cross-bred gilts generally cycle sooner than purebred stock.

Environmental influences may also be manipulated to cause the early development of puberty. In total confinement systems gilts raised in pens with four or more penmates mature faster sexually than gilts that are individually tethered or not allowed to interact with other gilts at all. It is recommended to exclude mature boars from gilt pens well before the females attain puberty as this can delay its arrival, but conversely, if boars are mixed in close to, but before the normal period in which puberty is developed it comes on sooner than it normally would.

Breeding Systems

Hand Breeding

In hand breeding, the female is always kept apart from the male until she is recognized to be in heat. She is then let into his pen to be bred if he is alone and there is enough room, or they are moved to a separate breeding pen. This is the most common system with purebred cattle, thoroughbred horses, and pigs. Mares must be hobbled when hand bred in order to prevent them from injuring the stallion by bucking or kicking as he mounts.

Hand breeding allows the farmer to observe matings closely and to assist if he or she needs to. The possibility of a chance mating doesn't arise because you are choosing which male to breed which female. It enables a good sire, whose blood you want to disseminate through your herd, to breed more females than he would be able to under range or pasture conditions. Accurate record keeping is improved, and most importantly of all, you are able to verify that breedings are in fact taking place. This last point seems self-evident, but on a large ranch oftentimes it is not that easy from a management standpoint to determine if estrus females have been bred and settled, especially if you have a fly over the herd or spend a couple of hours roaring along in a four-wheel drive truck just to sight them.

The major drawbacks to hand breeding are the time and labor involved, especially if your herd is very big or spread out. In spite of the increased time and cost it is the best method for a small operation or a farm of any size that bases its reputation and products on herd records and is concerned about reproductive efficiency.

Breeding Crates and Chutes

Breeding crates are used when breeding a gilt with a full-grown boar that would be too large for her to support during the mount, when using a small boar on a large, mature sow, or when using an old or lame boar. The crate can be adjusted to absorb the full-grown boar's weight, immobilize the sow, or allow a small boar to mount a larger sow by use of an inclined ramp. Also, by use of the ramp an old or lame boar may be able to breed well past its normal length of active service.

The breeding chute provides the same function in cattle.

Corral and Pen Breeding

Corral breeding is used with horses if hand breeding is not possible because of space or labor limitations. The estrous mare and stud are turned into a strongly fenced corral to mate. The owner or manager stays out of sight of the animals and does not interfere with the breeding. This is a much less desirable system than hand breeding because of the possibility of injury to valuable stock and the manager's inability to assist with the mount.

Pen breeding is the same system applied to pigs, confinement sheep, and goat operations. The reasons for using it are the same; however, because of the animals' size you are able to get into the pen to help out, but it still isn't as comfortable or as safe for all involved as hand breeding.

Pasture Breeding

In this breeding method, usually favored by those farmers who run a commercial herd and don't need breeding records or individual control of matings, the male is turned in with the females he is supposed to service just for the breeding season or he runs with them year round. This is a common system with beef cattle, sheep, and goats. It also requires little labor and time. Yet, to gain these savings you must give up the assurance that your females have been bred. The other disadvantage is that the male's breeding efficiency goes down because he will often repeatedly mount the same female. Because you are not able to control the frequency of mating in order to conserve the male's strength and sex drive this breeding system can lead to the temporary sterility of an overworked stud.

Artificial Insemination

Artificial insemination is a technique in which the semen of male sires is collected for insemination of females. The males mount a dummy female and ejaculate into an artificial vagina. The semen is then diluted and has an antibacterial agent, such as penicillin, streptomycin, or polymixin, added. It is then mixed with glycerin and frozen in liquid nitrogen to -320° F [-196° C] for storage or transport. Once the semen is thawed out it must be used immediately as the sperm's viability begins to decrease rapidly.

The amount of semen necessary to inseminate a female of the species is measured into a plastic pipette (a long, thin tube) called a *straw* that has been designed to pass through the vagina and lock into the cervix (in sows) or just penetrate the cervical canal, barely passing into the uterus (in cows). The semen is then deposited by the inseminator (if they are conscientious) in about the time it takes for the male to normally ejaculate.

When artificially inseminating a cow the inseminator puts on a long plastic or rubber glove that reaches up his or her arm almost to the shoulder. They cup their hand, holding their fingers together at the tips and force it into the cow's anus. The cow immediately and involuntarily defecates. The feces are scooped out and the hand is reinserted in the rectum, moving forward carefully each time the cow relaxes its wave-like muscular contractions. With their fingers downward the inseminator feels their way along the top wall of the vaginal canal until he or she reaches the cervix. It should feel like a series of hard rings. The insemi-nator grasps the cervix with his or her fingers so that when the straw is inserted through the vagina and either into or through the cervix, depend-ing on the species, the inseminator will be able to feel when he or she has reached the right spot to deposit the semen (see Figure 97).

Never attempt to artificially inseminate unless you have taken a training course from one of the reputable semen or breeder sales com-panies and know what you are doing, but by all means take the course and learn how to do it! If you do your own inseminating, always maintain the strict sterility of your equipment and make sure that the semen is stored at the correct temperature. More cows go unbred because of manage-ment errors than for any other reason.

The advantages of artificial insemination are myriad. If you have ever bred your cows with a dairy bull you know what unpredictable, powerful, self-willed, and worst of all, playful animals they are. And I am sure you've heard stories about how cute, lovable "Ferdinand," who was as meek as a newborn kitten, suddenly got a hankering for "Old Bess" and was renamed "Tornado" after he went straight through his pen, you, and the side of the barn to get to her. They aren't just stories and you sure don't want it to happen to you. Besides being dangerous to keep a sire, it is expensive in time, labor, feed, housing, and worry.

Through artificial insemination (AI) you can pick and choose any sire you want, living, or dead, giving you the chance to make real genetic progress in your herd. Because the sire you select has a documented breeding record based on what his daughters have done, you have a good idea of what you're getting before you pay for it. Your chances of a nasty surprise, like paying a fancy stud fee for a big, virile-looking stallion that turns out to be sterile, or a bull that gives your cow a venereal disease such as vibriosis, are close to nonexistent.

There are some disadvantages to artificial insemination that need to be recognized and remembered:

1. Not all inseminators have the same skill (ask around, both good and bad news travel fast).
2. The inseminator must be contacted as soon as animals come into heat.
3. Since you are working with a very busy man or woman (if they are any

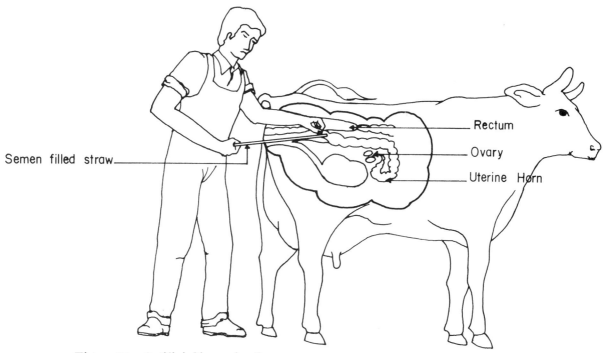

Figure 97. Artificial insemination.

kind of inseminator) heat detection must be first-class.
4. If you do your own insemination the semen must be stored at the proper temperature with special equipment which must be maintained in absolutely sterile condition.

The last word on AI is that it is practical, cheap, and, if used properly, can make your job a lot easier and more enjoyable.

When to Breed Your Animals

The First Time

Beef heifers should be bred to calve as 2-year-olds (24–27 months). This means that in a temperate zone you can safely breed them to a bull that sires small calves, such as an Angus, once they have reached at least 600–650 pounds (and are in good shape), depending on the breed, and are at least 13–14 months of age. In the tropics the first breeding should be at least 4–5 months later if your cattle are a Zebu type (Zebu, Brahma, Santa Gertrudis, etc.).

Dairy heifers that are well grown should be bred, on the average, at 14–16 months. (See the following "Breeding Guide for First-Calf Dairy Heifers.") At this point they are strong, growing well, and will have no trouble producing a healthy calf and reaching their full milking potential. If bred younger, calving problems and/or decreased milk production are real possibilities. If bred older these heifers won't make you as much money.

Mares shouldn't be bred before reaching 3 years of age. If they are bred as 2-year-olds there is a risk of permanent harm being done them

BREEDING GUIDE FOR FIRST-CALF DAIRY HEIFERS

Breed	Age at First Service (in months)	Weight at First Service (in pounds)
Jersey	14–17	500–600
Guernsey	15–18	550–650
Ayrshire	16–19	600–700
Holstein	16–20	800–900
Brown Swiss	17–20	800–900

Adapted from Bailey, *Veterinary Handbook for Cattlemen,* fifth edition, 1980, p. 200.

and the foals because neither animal's nutritional requirements will be met.

Ewe lambs should be bred in the next breeding season after they are at least 1 year old and weigh from 85–100 pounds. This will have them dropping their first lamb at close to 2 years old. Goat does are treated just like ewes and should also be bred to produce their first kid at 2 years.

Gilts can be bred at either their first or second heat if in good physical shape and if they weigh close to 220 pounds. This will have them farrowing at about a year of age (between 11 and 13 months).

After Giving Birth

Cows should not be bred back after freshening (giving birth) for 60 days to give them time to build up their nutritional levels after the drain of growing a healthy calf and a heavy lactation.

Mares are bred back on the second heat after foaling, usually between 25–30 days after giving birth. It's a good policy to wait until the 2nd heat because many mares have birth-related discharges or infections following foaling and are very liable to vaginal or uterine infection when serviced at their first heat.

Ewes raised in temperate zones are normally seasonal breeders, except for Finnsheep, Polypays, American Merinos, Debouillet, Delaine Merinos, Rambouillet, Tunis, Dorsets, and some crossbreds which will breed out of season. Those breeds that are seasonal breeders have to wait, of course, until the next breeding season before being bred back after lambing. Nonseasonal breeders in the temperate zones and all breeds in the tropics should be rested 45–60 days before breeding back. Goats should be treated like sheep. Sows are rebred at the first heat after their piglets have been weaned.

How Frequently Can a Sire Be Used for Breeding?

Beef Bulls

Beef bulls younger than 1 year of age, although capable of breeding, should never be used because of the unproven and questionable viability of their semen and the very real possibility of injuring their penises while attempting to mount a cow larger than them. Once bulls attain yearling status they can be used in hand-breeding operations but should be held back from range or pasture breeding until becoming 2-year-olds.

In general, bulls are able to breed productively in hand breeding and chute systems up to and beyond 10 years of age; on the range or pasture, 6–7 years is the average upper limit.

The following "Bull Service Guide" is meant to give you an idea of the total number of annual breedings permissible by age group in both hand and pasture breeding set-ups. Breedings in both groups should be spread out evenly during the year to give the bull time to rest and rebuild his strength. Don't cram all of a bull's services for the year into a few weeks; the only crop you will reap will be a sterile, possibly permanently damaged animal. The total number of services per year is lower for all age groups on pasture compared to hand breeding, because the bull is stressed much more. A good bull-to-cow ratio on pasture or range is 1:20–25.

BULL SERVICE GUIDE

Age Group (years)	Hand Breeding (services/yr)	Pasture Breeding (services/yr)
Less than 1 year	0	0
1	10–15	0
2	25–30	20–25
3	40–50	30–35
4	50–60	40–50

Adapted from Ensminger, *Animal Science,* seventh edition, 1977, p. 375.

Dairy Bulls

Dairy bulls are not used for breeding until 12–15 months old, except for very big, mature animals, and even then not at all before 10 months, and only sparingly afterward. Until reaching 18 months bulls are used a maximum of twice a week only over short periods of time. Mature bulls over 18 months may be bred up to 60 times a year, but spread out evenly to maintain their strength and to avoid temporary sterility. These mature bulls are used for service a maximum of 4 times a week during short periods not to exceed more than 2 weeks at a time.

Stallions

Stallions vary tremendously by health, breed, temperament, and hence, service ability. However, as a general rule, because of their calmer nature draft stallions are able to breed more frequently than light horse breeds. The only recommended breeding technique for horses is hand breeding, although corral breedings must occasionally be done for time, space, or labor considerations. Corral breeding is potentially dangerous for both animals and does not allow the manager to assist during service. In natural conditions horses are violent breeders, which is one of the reasons why mares are hobbled in hand breeding; but this isn't possible in the corral.

Most mature stallions are limited to a maximum of one service per day, 6 days a week, with 1 day off to rest, over short periods. Some very strong, mature stallions are able to serve twice a day, again with at least 1 day of rest per week. The best times for twice a day service are early in the morning and late in the afternoon. Both light and heavy breeding schedules have to be planned well to not conflict with eating. Service on an empty or light stomach is better for the digestion and sex drive.

Stallions are very long-lived if they receive the proper care and nutrition. Often a mature stallion will maintain enough virility and sufficient sex drive to continue serving mares into his 20s, albeit at a reduced frequency compared with his early years.

STALLION SERVICE GUIDE

Age Group (years)	Hand Breeding (services/yr)	Service Limit
1	0	0
2	10–15	2–3/week
3		
typical	20–40	1/day
Thoroughbreds	20–25	1/day
Standardbreds	25–30	1/day
4		
typical	30–60	2/day
Thoroughbreds	30–40	2/day
Standardbreds	40–50	2/day
5–17		
typical	80–100	2/day
draft breeds	100	2/day
18 and up	20–40	1/day

Adapted from Ensminger, *Animal Science,* seventh edition, 1977, p. 969.

Rams

Most sheep ranches are pasture or range operations. This calls for a lower ewe/ram ratio than can be used on the more labor intensive hand breeding farms. On rough range there should be three rams for every 100 ewes. Whether you have a big flock or a small one, whether they are run on pasture, range, backyard, or in confinement, you should use strong, mature rams 2 years and older for breeding. These rams will nicely serve 35–50 ewes each on good pasture or range and more (up to 75) on intensively run hand-breeding farms where they are separated from the ewes.

With good nutrition and supplemental feeding a vigorous ram should be breeding your ewes until he is 6–7 years old. On the range, where supplemental feeding is the exception to the rule and rams get worn out quickly through dominance fights, overbreeding, and poor nutrition, they will last only a couple of years at the best.

Yearling lambs can be used in a pinch but should be bred lightly (20–25 ewes a year) to continue their own growth and not be set back by overwork.

Goat Bucks

Goats should be treated much like rams. Bucks mature sexually at different rates depending on breed, climatic zone, and level of nutrition. Most produce viable sperm by at least 5-6 months, though I once heard a story of a precocious 3-month-old that successfully bred an older doe. Bucks and does should always be separated at 3 months, just in case an overly mature buck kid should appear in your herd. Put your young bucks to work serving does at 6 months. If they don't show signs of a healthy sexual appetite and don't impregnate estrous does, slaughter or sell them right away. There is no sense in giving them a free ride if they can't breed, for that is their sole function.

Boars

Young, well-grown boars are used for breeding (very sparingly) starting at 8 months of age. From 8-12 months they can be used once a day with a maximum of 5 matings a week. This is an extreme upper limit as it is only recommended to use them for a total of 25 matings in their 1st year of service. One-year-old boars and older may be used a maximum of twice a day with a total of 50 services per year.

With good care and nutrition a virile boar should be able to service your females up to 8 years of age with no problems. More normally, producers use a boar until he is 4-5 years old and then bring on a younger one. One of the biggest limitations to boar longevity, and their continuing ability to serve estrous females, is their feet. Pay close attention to foot rot and sore and crippled feet, especially in total confinement systems where the animals are on concrete all the time.

Prepare Your Sheep for Breeding

Trim Their Feet

Feet are usually the last thing producers check, if they do at all. Before breeding season is a good time for preventive foot maintenance, but make sure you trim them twice a year as a matter of course and examine them more frequently.

Sheep have two claws on their feet that, when properly trimmed or worn down by exercise, they should be able to stand on squarely with their weight evenly distributed. This means that the horn around the edge of the hoof must be trimmed with a knife or shears until it is even (level) with the sole (see Figure 98 a and b). Don't let them grow out too far in the front or they'll start to curl. If you don't keep them cut back, count on having sore-legged, limping stock that won't breed well.

If, after trimming, there are still depressions or identations in the foot clean them out and cut the claws back a bit further, keeping them close to level with the sole. You should eliminate these potential trouble spots as soon as they appear; frequently they get stones wedged in them inflaming the foot, and collect feces and mud, causing foot rot.

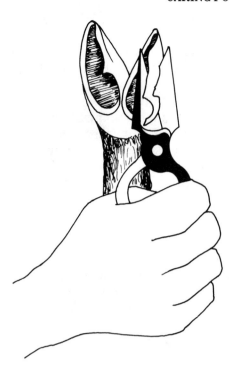

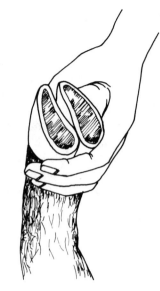

Figure 98b.   Trim your sheep's feet level (after).

Figure 98a.   Trim your sheep's feet level (before).

Shear the Rams

When the external temperature reaches 80° F (26.5° C) ram semen viability is reduced; as the temperature climbs to 90° F (32° C) they become impotent and often take weeks to regain their breeding ability. Therefore, when the breeding season in the temperate zones is in the summer (and in the tropics all year round) rams are sheared before being turned in with the flock. This causes them to perk up, become more active and interested in breeding, makes mating easier, and usually improves potency. Another trick to improve fertility in hot weather is to turn the ram in with the ewes at night and to separate them during the day. Not only does this reserve the cool of the night for breeding but enables you to supplement the ram's feed with a little grain during the day.

"Tagging" the Ewes

The caked mats of hair, dirt, and feces that build up around the ewe's tail are called tags and should be trimmed off before breeding season. Often these tags are the cause of unsuccessful copulation because they are so thick the ram is unable to penetrate the ewe with his penis during the mount.

Feeding to Breed

Beef Heifers

It is now common practice to raise beef heifers to calve as 2-year-olds, preferably around 30 months. In order to accomplish this feat, which entails the growing of a healthy calf by a still immature and developing mother, young heifers have to be fed quite well. Our goal is to bring these animals along at an average daily weight gain of 1½ pounds from weaning until breeding (and at the same rate until midpregnancy). This is done by keeping them on abundant and nutritious pasture with a free-choice mineral supplement and salt. If pasture is deficient or of poor quality, feed 1–2 pounds of a protein supplement daily per head in whatever form you like (cubes or blocks), plus the mineral supplement and salt.

Beef Cows

Cows' nutritional requirements are not as severe as those of heifers. They are mature animals that have finished their own body growth and can therefore be fed all they want of a poorer quality pasture or roughage. However, the roughage (analyzed as dry matter) must contain at least 5.9 percent total protein. If it doesn't, feed 1–2 pounds of a protein supplement. Always provide free-choice salt and a mineral supplement.

Be careful of overfeeding beef cattle since excess fat will be deposited around the reproductive tract. This lowers fertility, hinders conception, and can cause problems in calving.

Weaned to 3-Year-Old Beef Bulls

Weaned bulls up to 3 years of age need to be well fed in order to meet the nutrient requirements of their growing bodies and to develop the fertility demanded of them. With a good feeding schedule and plenty of exercise on pasture they should be ready for occasional breeding at 15 months.

If young bulls are used for breeding when pasture is limited or poor, if they are serving the upper limit of cows for their age group, or if they are breeding during drought conditions they need to be supplemented with extra grain. Don't cut costs here or you may permanently damage a fine bull. After finishing breeding for the year a 1-year-old bull gets his grain ration upped to 6 pounds, in addition to the good quality roughage he continues to receive.

Mature Beef Bulls

Mature bulls mixed in with the cows for the summer need no supplemental feeding if the pasture is high-quality mixed legume grass. In the winter they get 3–5 pounds of grain and 1 pound of protein supplement

YOUNG BULL FEEDING GUIDE

Age	Daily Gain (in pounds)	Feed as % Of Body Wt (each day)	Feed	Protein Supplement (each day)
Weaning– 15 months	2½	2½%	3–5 pounds of grain and roughage.	2 pounds
15 months– 3 years	2–2¼	2–2¼%	Keep increasing the % of roughage and decreasing the % of grain	2 pounds

(32%) daily, along with as much good protein hay as they want. Always provide salt and a mineral supplement free-choice. Two months before the start of breeding season the protein supplement goes to 1¼–1½ pounds daily depending on how much the animal needs to be built up. Always make sure your bulls are exercising and that they've got a big enough field to really move around in—your calf crop depends on the soundness of their condition.

Dairy Heifers

Calves are weaned at 4-6 weeks, by which time they should be eating 1-2 pounds of starter concentrate a day. For the first week after weaning they should consume an 18% protein starter and all the good quality hay (first or second-cut green, leafy legume hay), they want to stimulate rumination. This is continued until 16-24 weeks of age; however, the starter is limited to a maximum intake of 5 pounds per day. If your hay is poor quality the maximum concentrate level is upped to 6-8 pounds per day.

At 16-24 weeks the 18 percent ration is changed to a normal 16 percent milking (lactation) ration, with the hay still fed free-choice. At 32 weeks the 16 percent concentrate is cut out and the heifers are only fed hay or silage unless its quality or their condition call for the continuation of the grain. Two weeks before giving birth heifers are started in at 4 pounds of grain a day and slowly built up so that by calving time they are consuming 6-10 pounds daily.

Dairy Cows

Once cows calve, approximately 60 days pass before they are bred back. This is a period (which lasts until 10 weeks after calving) when the animal physically cannot consume as much energy in its feed as it puts out in the milk it produces. The difference in energy comes from what the cow has stored up before calving.

Starting 2 weeks before giving birth cows are fed 4 pounds of grain per day so that by calving time they are eating 6–10 pounds of grain daily to get them ready for milking. After they have calved a general rule for feeding is that their ration should be 60 percent concentrates and 40 percent roughage, but this is adjusted to account for feed prices. The exact weights and types of feeds should be determined by individual milking ability, ingredient availability and price, feeding system, and other factors.

Dairy Bulls

Young dairy bulls are fed like heifers, though supplemented a little more than they are. Mature bulls are fed the same percent protein concentrate ration as the milkers are on the basis of a half pound of grain for every 100 pounds of body weight. Bulls of all ages are offered salt and a mineral supplement fed free-choice and must receive plenty of exercise to keep from getting fat, sluggish, and impotent.

Mares

For the first 3 months after foaling a mare consumes 2 percent of its weight daily in dry matter (approximately 22 pounds), of which 45–55 percent is concentrate and the rest is roughage. These percentages are rough guides and will fluctuate due to the mare's condition, the amount of milk she produces, and the quality of her hay or the grass she is pastured on. Plan on a 14 percent average crude protein level for her ration and always provide salt and a mineral supplement free-choice.

Stallions

Stallions should have their normally good forage supplemented with a concentrate 2–3 weeks before the start of breeding season. Then, as breeding begins, concentrate intake should be increased to 1 pound daily per each 100 pounds of body weight for the duration of the season. Make sure the roughage is green, leafy, and that it tests at 10 percent protein or better; the whole ration (including the roughage portion) should be formulated at 14 percent on a dry weight basis. Always provide salt and a mineral supplement fed free-choice.

Ewes

For several weeks before and after breeding ewes are grazed on good quality pasture containing grass and legumes or fed an early cut, green, leafy grass–legume hay mixture. If grazed on only leguminous pasture their lamb crop will be smaller than normal because the high estrogen (a female sex hormone) levels found in legumes will reduce fertility. In addition to roughage they should receive a small amount of grain each day from weaning to breeding in order to put on a little weight but not so much that they get fat. Provide salt and a mineral supplement, free-choice.

Rams

Rams are grazed on good quality pasture before breeding season or are fed a comparable quality hay, but at a higher level than ewes. If their condition warrants it they can be beefed up (but not to the point of becoming fat) with a small grain ration before and during the breeding season. This is easiest to do if they are separated from the ewes during the day and fed separately. Provide salt and a mineral supplement, free-choice.

Goat Does

Doe kids are fed 4 pints of milk a day along with mature, leafy green pasturage or hay from weaning until 4 months. In the 4th month the milk is cut to 3 pints; in the 5th month it goes to 2 pints; in the 6th month it drops to 1 pint, and 2 weeks later the milk stops altogether. At 26 weeks doe kids are fed a diet consisting entirely of roughage (but never let them graze wet pasture or consume high-moisture silage) that can be supplemented with a little concentrate—up to a maximum of 1 pound/day—if the roughage is poor quality. Roughage, root crops, and greens will carry them to first breeding. Always provide salt and a mineral supplement free-choice.

Goat Bucks

Young bucks are fed just like doe kids, except they receive an extra pint of milk per day until the 4th month. After cutting out the milk, as described above, they are fed at a little higher level than the does. If pasture or roughage is poor and your bucks look scruffy give them a small grain ration daily (⅖ pound per animal) to tone them up. Coming into the breeding season they get ⅓–½ pound of grain per day per animal, but this must be adjusted to keep them from getting fat. Provide salt and a mineral supplement, free-choice.

Mature bucks need more roughage than does and should get 1–2 pounds of grain a day unless they start to look fat. Keep them exercising, it will help them become more vigorous in their breeding.

Gilts and Sows

After reaching 175–200 pounds gilts have their feed restricted to 5 pounds daily of pregestation concentrate until they come into heat. Let mature sows, after their piglets have been weaned, balance their own nutrient needs by unrestricted consumption but drop them down from a 16 percent protein lactation ration to a 12 percent protein pregestation ration.

Boars

Young, growing boars of up to 120 pounds get a high protein grower ration (18 percent protein) but are limited to 5–5½ pounds of concentrate per day. Boars from 120–250 pounds (on a 16 percent protein ration) and mature boars 250 pounds and up (on a 14 percent protein ration) are limited to 4¼ pounds of concentrate per day. These figures are supplemented by feeding roughage.

When feeding a complete feed without an additional roughage young boars can receive up to 9 pounds/day; mature boars get 5-7 pounds per day. Always keep boars in good trim, never fat nor skinny. These feeding guidelines must be adjusted for breed differences, individual temperament, humidity, temperature, type of housing, and stress.

Rabbits

Growing and unbred does and bucks need feed with 12-15 percent protein and close to 22 percent fiber. Generally, green, good quality, leafy legume hay fed free-choice is enough to maintain mature breeding animals. If they need fleshing out and/or the hay is not good quality, supplement them with 2 ounces of feed pellets daily for each 8 pounds of body weight. Mature bucks that are serving does get 4-6 ounces of pellets daily or unlimited good hay plus 2 ounces of pellets.

Flushing

Flushing is a widespread practice in which the feed of ewes and sows is increased a few weeks before breeding, and then is let down gradually to normal levels following service in ewes, and cut back immediately in sows. It quickly gets females into good condition for breeding, causes them to come into heat together, and most importantly, they shed more ova than normal. The effects of this last point can be convincingly shown in increased lambing and farrowing rates—up to 25 percent more offspring.

Sheep farmers claim that flushing should be done somewhere between 2-3 weeks before breeding, but the most cost-effective results show up when started 17 days before service. Ewes are put on good quality green pasture and supplemented with a quarter pound of grain the first day. Slowly build them up to three-quarters of a pound per ewe per day within a week. Continue feeding at this level until you reach day 17.

The ewes are bred on their second heat after starting the flushing, during which they produce more ova than normal and have an increased tendency to twin. After reaching the 17th day the grain supplement is slowly cut back to nothing over 2 weeks.

Flushing gives best results in mature ewes if done towards the beginning or end of the breeding season. Ewe lambs don't respond well to flushing and it can further lower an already low conception rate in fat ewes.

Sows are flushed for 2 weeks before breeding, based on age and weight, with a 14-16 percent protein level concentrate. Gilts are fed 2½ pounds per each 100 pounds of body weight; sows receive 1½ pounds of concentrate per each 100 pounds of body weight. Once both gilts and sows have been bred the second time (both gilts and sows are serviced 2 days in a row during their heats to assure maximum fertilization) they are reduced the same day to a gestation ration.

Male Breeding Behavior

Bulls

Bulls quickly locate cows in heat and sniff and lick their vulvas. Since the cow often turns to sniff the bull's penis, they circle with each one's head facing the other's rear. The bull rubs his head on the cow's rump as he sniffs and licks her. This causes his penis to start dripping. Frequently the male butts the cow in the rump several times in a row to see if she will accept his mount. If she stands still in the mating position with her tail held to the side, sometimes bellowing repeatedly, the bull rests his head on her back and lunges forward in a practice mount. He does this several times before finally mounting in earnest, cradling her sides with his front legs, resting his weight on her back, and penetrating her vulva and vagina with his penis. The actual mating lasts a second or less and the bull ejaculates as soon as he enters the cow. The ejaculation is usually so strong it looks like the bull leaps up. The bull's feet do, in fact, come off the ground.

Stallions

A mare in heat, in the presence of a stallion, squats and urinates frequently. This in turn causes the stallion to urinate on the same spots to mark them. The male sniffs and licks the mare's vulva and bites her neck and back. If she is receptive to the stallion the mare takes the mating position: she stands motionless, stretches her hind legs backwards, lifts her tail up and to the side, and exposes her clitoris.

The stallion's penis is dripping a little by now and he attempts a few practice mounts. When he does mount the mare to mate he grasps her with his forelegs and rests his weight on her as described for the bull. Once the stallion has mounted he moves his pelvis back and forth rapidly several times to bring himself to erection. He enters the mare and passes through the vagina and cervix to the uterus, where he ejaculates. On the average, mating lasts 40 seconds.

Rams

The ram sniffs and licks the ewe's flanks and vulva. She responds by sniffing at his penis, causing them to turn around head to tail. The ewe bleats and is answered by the ram's courtship grunts. He approaches her from the rear by turning his head on its side and paws her hind leg with one of his fore legs. The ewe wags her tail rapidly, bleats, and assumes the immobile mating position. She turns her head back as if to watch the ram's practice mounts. He mounts, grasps her with his forelegs and moves his pelvis back and forth several times to bring himself to erection. Then he enters arching backward, as he ejaculates instantaneously.

Goat Bucks

The buck sniffs and licks the female's vulva; she sniffs at his penis and they turn in place, each one's head towards the other's genitals. The goat bleats often and is answered by the buck's gutteral grunts. When receptive the female stands motionless in the mating position and turns her head back toward the buck. He begins practice mounting. When the final mount takes place the buck rests his weight on the female's rump, thrusts his pelvis into her vulva to erect himself and penetrates her. He ejaculates almost immediately and arches his back and neck upward, like the ram. The mount lasts less than a second, the buck dismounts and immediately licks his penis.

Boars

The boar pokes the sow in the flanks with his snout and they grunt to each other with a gutteral chattering. They circle, sniffing each other's genitals, and switch to head to head "mock fights," in which they grind their teeth, salivate a frothy saliva which drips from their mouths and, jowl to jowl, try to push and shove each other with their heads (see Figure 99).

The sow pricks her ears up and forward, humps her back, and stands motionless when in the mating position. The boar usually mounts and dismounts several times before the final mount in which he moves his pelvis back and forth until the tip of his penis penetrates the sow's vulva. The boar enters the sow and alternates between active copulation, thrusting irregularly several times in succession, and resting. Many times during mating the sow will apparently start to walk away, especially when the boar is resting. This appears to stimulate him to fresh copulation and the sow once again stands immobile. The whole mating act takes up to 20 minutes, with the boar ejaculating into the cervix and uterus.

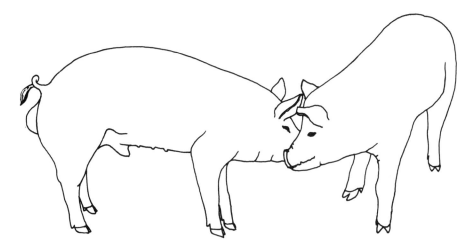

Figure 99.   Premounting behavior between a boar and a sow or gilt.

Anestrus

The term *anestrus* means the lack of estrus. Since heat doesn't occur, the female is not receptive to the male, and breeding doesn't happen. In some cases this is a normal body reaction that has evolved to regulate breeding cycles, to conserve energy during periods of great stress, such as lactation, or as part of the aging process. In other cases anestrus indicates a deficiency of minerals, vitamins, or energy.

Freemartins

Heifers born twin to a bull, called *freemartins,* are usually permanently anestrus because they are sterile (90 percent of the time). While the twins develop in the uterus the fetal blood of the heifer and the bull normally circulates through both of their bodies. The male sex hormones, those chemicals which trigger the development and maintenance of male sexual characteristics and function, are secreted into the blood several weeks before the female sex hormones are. Since both the male and female blood systems are normally linked in twin calf fetuses, the male sex hormones circulate in the female's body and disrupt its normal sexual development. The result is that the freemartin develops the internal reproductive organs of both a male and a female. Neither set of organs works and although the heifer outwardly looks female, it is sterile.

Seasonal Anestrus

Seasonal anestrus is common to horses, sheep, and goats. It is what we called *seasonal breeding* earlier. There is a good deal of variation within each of these species: some breeds are seasonally anestrus, others are to some extent, and yet others are not at all. The environment also creates anestrus behavior—many seasonally anestrus breeds in the Temperate Zone become year-round breeders in the tropics and vice versa.

Lactational Anestrus

Anestrus caused by intense lactation is common in cattle and sheep. The severity and length of the condition are influenced by breed, amount of milk produced, number of young being nursed, the season in which birth took place, and how much the uterus has returned to normal after birth.

Ewes usually don't come back into heat until 2 weeks after their lambs have been weaned. A 5-7 week absence of heat after birth is normal. Cows with nursing calves have a longer anestrus period than cows that are being milked; very high-producing milk cows are more frequently anestrus than more moderate milkers. Poorly fed Brahma cows nursing calves during very hot weather are best known for becoming anestrus, but most beef breeds will stop developing estrus when nursing on low energy diets.

Nutritional Anestrus

Inadequate energy levels in feed formulation often produce anestrus in young, still maturing female animals. Older, more mature females are not stressed as much by low-energy rations. Anestrus can also be caused by deficiencies of vitamin A and E, phosphorus (in cows and ewes), and manganese (in cows and gilts).

19

PREGNANCY AND BIRTH

Pregnancy Check

It is important to know if your bred females have become pregnant in order to adjust your feeding schedules, identify breeding problems, and to be able to cull (remove from the herd) unproductive animals. When developing feeding programs it has to be taken on faith that all bred females are, in fact, pregnant (and must receive a gestation ration) until proven otherwise.

There is no sense investing the money on the feed needed to bring a just-bred pregnant cow to term if she isn't pregnant. Pregnancy checks remove a good deal of the hit-and-miss aspects from raising animals. Learn how to do them or pay your veterinarian to check your animals; either way you will save money, labor, and time.

How to Do It

If your cow doesn't come back into heat an average of 21 days after being bred chances are good that she is pregnant. It is very difficult to check if she is pregnant until 60 days after breeding, so assume she is and treat accordingly. At 60 days you can insert your hand and arm into the cow's rectum (after putting on a long plastic glove called an *obstetrical sleeve* and lubricating it with a nonirritating lubricant or mild soap and water) in an operation known as palpation (to explore by feeling).

The purpose of inserting your hand into the cow is to feel along its reproductive tract, which lies right under the rectum, to determine if there is a fetus in the uterus. If you anticipate being inside the cow for any length of time, which is common when you are first learning how to pregnancy check, turn the obstetrical sleeve inside out before starting so the plastic seam doesn't irritate the mucous membrane that lines the inside of the rectum.

Hold your fingers together at their tips and gently insert your hand and arm into the cow's rectum. This will probably cause the cow to immediately defecate. Don't worry, it's nothing personal, just an involuntary muscular reaction. Scoop out the feces. If you feel strong pressure against your arm stop and wait for the cow to relax her muscles. Be very careful as you move forward in the rectum (your hand, with your fingers together, should advance slowly and cautiously in a slight up-and-down, wavelike swimming motion). The rectal membrane is strong and elastic in design but will rupture with needlessly rough movements. It should feel slippery; if for any reason it feels rough or you experience friction, remove your arm. Friction is an indication that the membrane is seriously irritated and that you may be wearing through it. If this occurs, stop and wait for another day.

Feeling gently downward through the wall of the rectum, locate the cervix, which feels like a series of hard rings close together in a row. You should reach the cervix well before inserting your arm to the elbow. Follow the outline of the cervix forward to the front of the pelvis until you reach the uterus. If the cow is pregnant, at 2 months the uterus will be swollen with fluid and the fetus will be a couple of inches long, the size of a mouse (see Figure 100).

Pat the uterus very gently; it will feel like a balloon filled with water. As the fetus floats upward it will bump against your hand, then float downward and back up once again before bumping your hand a second time.

At 3 months the uterus, because of its increasing weight, sinks into the abdominal cavity and to locate it you have to reach down into it, over the front of the pelvis. If at this stage you can't find the cervix, don't worry, it is a good sign that the cow is indeed pregnant. At 90 days the fetus is the size of a good-sized rat; at 120 days it is the size of a cat.

Mares are palpated rectally, after being well restrained, between 30 and 45 days, as described for cows. Once locating the uterus follow the curve of each of its horns with your hand. If the mare is pregnant the fetus is usually found in the bottom third of one of the horns, normally the right one. The fetus feels like an oval swelling or bulge at the bottom of the horn, the size of a large grape at 30 days and that of an orange at 45 days.

Only cows and mares have a reproductive tract large enough to palpate rectally by hand. An ultrasonic test for pregnancy can be done in ewes, goats, and sows but is very expensive and can't be justified economically unless your pure-bred stock is exceedingly valuable.

Use a Palpation Chute for Pregnancy Checks

A palpation chute is easily made by slightly modifying an existing wooden or steel chute that is too narrow for the animal to turn around in. A solid wooden gate is slipped into the chute, from above or the side, in front of the animal. The gate should be high enough so that the animal can't easily see over it. If the animal is able to look over it or if the gate is made of poles or timbers the animal will try to jump it if it gets excited. A pole or timber is slipped low through the chute behind the animal to keep

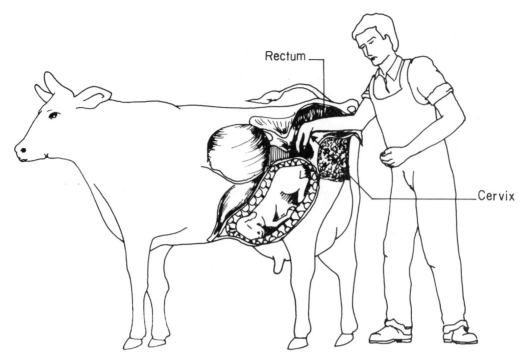

Figure 100.   How to check pregnancy.

it from backing up or kicking. Keep this pole or timber low enough to be able to get your arm out of the rectum in a hurry should the animal decide to lie down (see Figure 101).

Feeding for Pregnancy

First-Calf Beef Heifers

Since heifers are bred to calve for the first time as 2-year-olds, before having completed their growth, it is important to give them a ration formulated to continue their own development as well as that of their calf. However, it is necessary to prevent these young animals from fattening up after breeding or they will have problems at birth.

When heifers are first bred (at 600–650 pounds) until they calve, their average rate of gain should be between ¾–1 pound of body weight a day. This means they need to consume more than 1½ pounds of crude protein daily. This feeding schedule should have them weighing a minimum of 775 pounds with 4 months left before giving birth. In these final 4 months they are fed to gain 100–125 pounds and to be ready to calve at a minimum weight of 875 pounds (but try to bring them to term above this weight, if at all possible).

These growth rates can be adequately maintained on good quality pasture or hay (if feeding the latter supplement with vitamin A), with salt and a mineral supplement provided free-choice. If the roughage is poor quality feed a 48 percent protein supplement (1–2 pounds a day), or a pro-portionally larger quantity of a lower percentage supplement (for

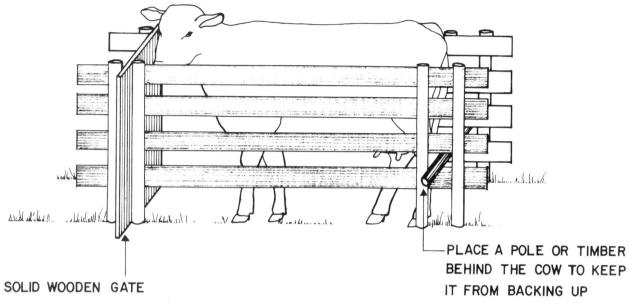

PLACE A POLE OR TIMBER BEHIND THE COW TO KEEP IT FROM BACKING UP

SOLID WOODEN GATE

Figure 101.   The palpation chute.

example, if you want to feed a 24 percent protein supplement you should offer the heifer 2-4 pounds/day). All protein supplements must contain vitamin A.

Second-Calf Beef Heifers

Second-calf heifers are fed for an average gain from weaning until birth of 1 pound a day. Once they have weaned their first calf (which should be done early, at 2-6 months, instead of the normal 7 months) until midpregnancy they are fed to gain an average of 1½ pounds per day. From midpregnancy until calving the daily gain is cut back to three-quarters of a pound. These gains can be made with good quality legume hay (with as much fed as the heifer will clean up) or pasturage. If the quality is poor then use a protein supplement (containing vitamin A) and always provide salt and a mineral supplement free-choice.

Mature Beef Cows

Dry cows, those that have stopped milking, need to gain 100-150 pounds of body weight before giving birth. This translates into a daily gain of one-half pound. Cows that are nursing calves need half again as much (50 percent more) energy and twice as much protein, phosphorus, and calcium in their feed as dry cows. This means that during the winter a dry pregnant cow could make as much gain on 18 pounds of a mixed grass-legume hay as a pregnant cow nursing a calf could make on 30 pounds of the same hay. Both rations would guarantee the animals' daily energy and protein requirements; of course, salt and a mineral supplement must be fed free-choice.

With mature cows, as with heifers, there are trade-offs between grass-legume hay, haylage (green chop), grain silages, grain, and protein supplements. For more detailed information the reader would do well to consult a recent edition of *Nutrient Requirements of Beef Cattle* edited by the National Research Council of the National Academy of Sciences in Washington, D.C.

DAILY DRY-FEED NEEDS OF MATURE PREGNANT BEEF COWS

Cow Stage	Body Condition	Dry-feed as a Percentage of Body Weight
Nursing	Poor	3⅜
	Average	3
	Good	2⅝
Dry	Poor	2¼
	Average	2
	Good	1¾

First-Calf Dairy Heifers and Mature Cows

By calving time heifers and mature cows have been built up to 6-10 pounds of grain per day to get them ready for a high level of milk production. After calving animals should be challenged to achieve high milking levels (the peak is reached 21-42 days after giving birth) by increasing their grain ration 1½ pounds a day to a maximum of 30-36 pounds daily.

Another feeding system that is widely followed is the feeding of grain in relation to milk produced, as seen in the following table:

Breed of Cattle	1 lb of Grain is Fed for Each Number of lbs of Milk Produced*	Grain Feeding Begins at What Level of Milk Production (in lbs.)
Jersey	1½	15–20
Guernsey	1½	15–20
Milking Shorthorn	1½	15–20
Red Poll	1½	15–20
Ayrshire	2	20–30
Brown Swiss	2	20–30
Holstein	2	20–30

*This is, of course, dependent on the price of milk relative to that of grain.

This is a general guide that can be followed until milk production reaches 80 pounds, then it becomes quite inaccurate.

Both of these graining systems are, at best, averages and estimates based on the typical cow. Since there is really no typical cow it would be foolish to blindly follow any feeding guide. A few basic rules on the amount of grain to feed, however, should be observed:

1. Base the amount of grain on how much milk your cows are able to produce—don't overfeed poor milkers or underfeed good ones.
2. The price of grain relative to what you receive for your milk must be carefully monitored at all times.

3. The price of good quality roughage must be calculated as a trade-off against grain.
4. Determine the availability of good quality roughage as compared to that of good quality grain.

This means that you have to adjust the amount of grain or concentrate you feed to each cow based on that animal's ability to produce, the cost trade-off between grain and roughage (but bear in mind that there are limits to how much hay and silage a cow can physically consume), and the value of the milk that an animal produces. As you challenge each cow it is essential to keep good records of the amount of milk and butter fat produced during which stage of the lactation based on what level of feeding. Following an evaluation of these records you will be able to vary feeding levels in order to give yourself the greatest return (milk, butterfat, and ultimately, income) on your investment (grain and roughage).

Roughage is the bulk of a dairy cow's diet. If only fed hay a cow will consume 2–3 pounds per every 100 pounds of body weight to a maximum of 3 percent of her weight. Corn silage can be substituted for dry hay at a ratio of 3 pounds to each pound of hay. Three pounds of good quality hay, such as a grass–legume mixture, must be fed to equal the energy content of 2 pounds of grain.

On a strictly forage diet cows are only able to produce 70 percent of the milk they are capable of producing when fed forage plus a concentrate or grain. The reason for this is that the cow's four-part stomach isn't sufficiently large enough to hold all the forage it would need to derive the energy necessary to milk to its true potential. Hence the need for grain: it contains more energy in a smaller mass than roughage. Our goal is to combine the two in a feeding ration that enables the cow to produce the most amount of milk and butterfat at the lowest cost.

Now we'll go back to the trade-off between forage and grain. Since you know, or can figure out, the maximum weight of roughage that each cow can consume daily (based on its body weight) and you have a rough guide of how many pounds of grain a cow milking at each level of production should receive, you can formulate a ration for each of your animals if you know their protein, energy, mineral, and vitamin requirements. At this point the reader is referred to several sources in order to learn how to balance rations: *Nutrient Requirements of Dairy Cattle* and the *Tables of Feed Composition*, both published by the National Academy of Sciences; chapter 18 of *Feeds and Nutrition* by Ensminger and Olentine (Ensminger Publishing); and chapter 41 of *Feeds and Feeding* by Cullison (Reston Publishing).

Dairy cattle are dried off (no longer milked) at different times before calving depending on their age and level of production. Heifers are dried off 60–65 days before calving; older cows are dried off 50–60 days before freshening. If a mature cow is a very high producer it should be dried off at 60–65 days, like heifers.

The dry period lets cows rest after the stress of milking, lets them build up their bodies to prepare for their next lactations, and helps them grow out healthy calves. The technique employed to dry cows off depends on their milking level. If they weren't producing much milk at the end of their lactation milking should stop altogether, the grain ration is discontinued, and their water reduced substantially. For those cows still producing decent amounts of milk at the end of their lactations, feed is changed from high to low energy, and grain and water are restricted. Continue milking them but taper it off quickly. Turn dry cows out on pasture or feed them medium quality hay (keep the energy down) and make sure they don't gain too much weight.

Mares

Several days before a mare foals her grain is cut back and the ration should become more laxative. Include some bran or linseed meal to keep her from getting constipated. She should be allowed to drink up to half a bucket of lukewarm water in small amounts just before birth and again after giving birth.

The mare's first meal after foaling, which in quantity is one half of the size of her normal ration, is a mixture of bran with a little oats or oatmeal soaked in warm water and fed as a mash; also offer some hay. The next day the amount of oats is increased and the bran is decreased. This continues for a week, along with a lot of very good quality legume hay. The mare slowly receives more and more oats if her appetite and milk production warrant it. In 7–10 days she is back to eating a normal-sized ration.

Don't rush your animal to consume too much grain during this first week and a half. If too much oats are fed after foaling the mare's milk production increases greatly and the next thing you know you've got a colicky foal with scours. If the mare foals on green nutritious pasture she will have no trouble controlling her own feed consumption to produce just the right amount of milk during this critical period.

Lactation stresses the mare and causes her nutritional requirements to increase for protein, energy, minerals (especially calcium and phosphorus), and vitamins (either carotene or vitamin A). These nutritional needs increase markedly in the last 3 months before foaling when the fetus makes its most active growth.

The lactating mare from foaling to 3 months is fed a ration containing 12.5 percent crude protein, approximately 55 percent of which, by weight, is a good quality mixed legume—grass hay (the best legume is alfalfa cut when 10 percent of it is in bloom) and 45 percent, by weight, is a 16 percent crude protein concentrate. For the next 1–3 months, depending on when her foal is weaned at 4–6 months after birth, the mare receives a ration containing 11 percent crude protein, of which 70 percent, by weight, is a good quality legume-grass hay and 30 percent, by weight, is a 12 percent crude protein concentrate. From weaning until just before foaling, the pregnant mare receives a ration with 11 percent crude protein that contains approximately 75 percent, by weight, good legume-grass hay and 25 percent, by weight, of a 12 percent crude protein concentrate.

If pregnant mares are run on good quality legume-grass pasture the grain portion of their feed ration can be figured at ¾–1 pound for each 100 pounds of body weight daily.

During the entire lactation and pregnancy mares must be provided with abundant water, salt, and a mineral supplement (containing calcium and phosphorus) fed free-choice. Don't stint on the exercise, it is good for both the mare and the normal development of the fetus. Pregnant draft horses can be lightly worked up to a week before foaling.

Ewes

Ewes should be run on good quality legume-grass pasture until lambing. The pasturage will be enough, along with salt and a mineral supplement, to satisfy their nutritional requirements until 6 weeks before lambing. At this point they receive ½-¾ pound of grain daily (preferably a mixture in equal proportions of wheat, oats, and corn) all the way until giving birth. The total weight gain during pregnancy should be 20-30 pounds, so adjust the graining to keep ewes on schedule. They should be neither too fat nor a bag of bones at lambing time. If your animals are run on range, feeding this grain supplement will be impractical; use range cubes or protein supplement pellets instead.

At all times ewes must have access to salt and a mineral supplement fed free-choice. Give your animals enough pasture to keep their body tone up through plenty of exercise; animals raised in confinement housing also need exercise every day if you are to prevent lambing difficulties.

Goat Does

Does have their overall rations decreased and the high fiber roughage portion of them increased after birth and for the next 3-4 days. Then, because does are high milking animals, they must be given enough good quality feed to get the job done to the best of their genetic ability. Having the right tools (excellent forage and grain) makes their work possible.

Good-quality legume-grass hay is the basis of their ration; the better the quality, the less amount of grain that must be fed when prices are high. However, like the cow, the doe produces milk at the high point of her lactation with a net energy deficit. She can't eat enough energy-containing foods to equal the amount of energy she puts out in her milk. So from our (the producers') standpoint we want to fill her up with as much high-energy feed as is physically possible and economically justifiable during the peak of her lactation. Understandably, challenge feeding, as we discussed in dairy cattle, is also the norm with viable goat herds.

Challenge grain feeding in goats is related to milking potential, stage of lactation, the cost of grain relative to the price of milk, the cost of grain relative to high-quality legume forage, and the availability of both grain and forage. In general, milking does are fed 1½-2 pounds of grain a day, in addition to forage. But a more relevant guide is provided by the following table:

Stage of Lactation	lbs of Grain Consumed: lbs of Milk Produced	lbs of Top Quality Legume Hay/100 lbs of Body Wt (daily)
Early	1:3	2½
Peak	1–1½:3	2½
Late	1:4–5	2½

By drying off time (at least 56 days before kidding) does are down to one half pound of grain daily. Dry your milkers off by restricting their water intake, cutting off the grain entirely, and by reducing the energy level of their forage. If they are still milking well milk them less and less frequently. Try to upset them and disturb their normal habits at milking time so they won't let their milk down, until they stop altogether over a week period. As you milk this final week, keep stripping them out completely as before. You will be able to completely stop milking when production drops below 2 pounds at each milking.

If their milk production is already low by the end of lactation (below 4 pounds a day) just stop milking the day you want to dry them off. They'll bleat and be uncomfortable for a day and then their udders will deflate like old balloons.

At the very end of the dry period, 2–3 weeks before dropping their kid(s), does should be fed sappy root crops, if they are available. They are good as a tonic and bring on an abundant milk flow. Good sources of these are kale, mangolds, turnips, sugar beets, comfrey, and carrots.

Sows

Gilts and sows are fed reduced amounts of a 14–16 percent farrowing ration 4–5 days before and after farrowing. Feed during this period should be laxative in nature (it should contain bran, oats, and possibly, sugar beet pulp) and bulky in texture. The reason for this change in diet is to clean the animals' intestinal tracts out to facilitate farrowing and to prepare them for the high-energy ration they will need for lactation.

Following these few days after farrowing sows are put on a 16 percent protein lactation ration and are allowed to self-limit their own consumption. Piglets are weaned at 3–4 weeks, at which point sows are limited to 4 pounds per day of a 12 percent gestation ration. Alternatively, they can be fed 8 pounds every 2nd day or 12 pounds every 3rd day as a labor-saving measure. Don't allow pregnant sows to consume more than the recommended daily feed level from weaning until 4–5 days before farrowing or they will be too fat at birth. An increased mortality at farrowing is a common result.

If animals are fed at recommended levels gilts will gain 70 pounds (around nine-tenths of a pound each day) and sows will gain 90 pounds (approximately seven-tenths of a pound daily) during pregnancy.

Rabbit Does

Since rabbits change their level of consumption in order to balance their energy needs at the different stages of their lives, the easiest feeding system for producers is to select the proper complete feed for the stage the doe is in (lactation or gestation) and provide enough for your animals to self-feed. As a general rule 10-pound lactating does consume just over 8 ounces a day, 5-pound gestating does eat 4 ounces daily and 10-pound gestating does usually consume around 7 ounces per day.

Lactating does are fed a complete feed containing 17 percent protein and 12–14 percent fiber until their bunnies are weaned at 6–8 weeks. From weaning until the last 10 days before kindling (giving birth) does are fed rations with 15 percent protein and 14–16 percent fiber. During the final 10 days before giving birth does are upped to a 17 percent protein ration in order to provide the nutrients the fetuses need in the final third of pregnancy, which is their fastest growth period.

GESTATION TABLE

Species	Breed	Length of Pregnancy (days)
Cattle	Aberdeen-Angus	281
	Ayrshire	278–79
	British Friesian	282
	Brown Swiss	290–91
	Charolais	289
	Guernsey	283–84
	Hereford	285
	Holstein-Friesian	278–79
	Jersey	279
	Red Poll	285
	Shorthorn	282
	Simmental	289
	Swedish Friesian	281–82
	Swedish Red & White	283–84
	Zebu	285
Horse	Draft breeds	333–45
	Light breeds	330–37
Sheep	Columbia	148–49
	Finnsheep	144–45
	Hampshire	144–45
	Karakul	151
	Lincoln	146–49
	Merino	150–51
	Rambouillet	150–51
	Romanov	144–45
	Romney	146–49
	Southdown	144–45
	Targhee	148–49
Goat		143–57 (150 average)
Pig		112–15 (114 average)
Rabbit		30–33

The gestation period for first-calf heifers is usually 2 days shorter than the breed average. Bull calves are normally carried 1 day longer in a full-term pregnancy than heifer calves.

Getting Ready for Birth

Cattle

Pregnant beef cows are separated from the rest of the herd and turned onto clean, fresh pasture—preferably close to the farm or ranch—several days before calving. This will prevent injury from other cattle, give the soon-to-calve cows the seclusion they seek out naturally, and lets you keep a close eye on them.

When the weather doesn't permit calving outdoors a maternity pen 12 × 12 feet should be prepared by cleaning out and disinfecting an unused pen in an unheated barn. Bed it well with short-stemmed straw over at least 4 inches of dry sawdust or sand and make sure there is adequate lighting. Move the cow in several days before calving to get it used to its temporary quarters.

Dairy cows are always put in the maternity pen for calving regardless of the season, unless your herd is very large and you don't have space to accommodate all of your freshening cows at the same time. Even if space is limited it would be better to try and rearrange stalls rather than lose a calf because you weren't there to assist with the calving.

Mares

In good weather mares about to foal are moved to clean, well-drained pasture a week before giving birth. Only foaling mares are let onto this pasture, which is located close enough to the stable to be able to observe them from time to time. When the weather prevents foaling outside prepare a maternity stall 12 × 12 feet. Clean it out, disinfect it well (including walls and manger), and bed it down with at least 4 inches of sawdust or sand covered with a thick layer of short-stem straw. The stall must be in a quiet barn with good ventilation and adequate lighting. Remove all equipment, bins, and racks from the stall, leaving only the manger.

Ewes and Goat Does

If ewes are going to lamb in the late spring, summer, or early fall when the weather is balmy or warm it is a good idea to shear them 1 month before giving birth. This brings the ewe to lambing in a cleaner condition, which means the lamb is exposed to less dirt and germs, it makes it easier for you to assist with a problem birth, and helps the lamb find its mother's teats quicker.

If the weather or labor considerations preclude shearing, trim the wool from around your ewes' udders, flanks, and tails. This trimming is called *crutching;* when properly done your animals should look like the ewe in Figure 102.

The wool on the ewe's face is also trimmed off in an operation called, appropriately enough, *facing.* In breeds with heavy, thick wool on the face it helps ewes find and keep an eye on their lambs and lets them graze more efficiently. Light-wool breeds that have been faced look for shelter for themselves and their lambs in inclement weather, certainly a behavioral response worth encouraging.

If you anticipate lambing difficulty or the weather is cold, rainy, or rough move your ewe, especially if it is her first birth, to a lambing pen several days before the big event. The pen should measure 5 × 5 feet, be cleaned, disinfected, and well bedded with 4 inches of sawdust or sand covered with abundant short-stemmed straw. Make sure the lighting and

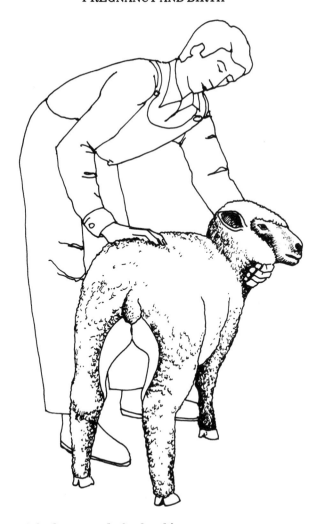

Figure 102.   A crutched ewe ready for lambing.

ventilation are good and that it is in a quiet spot.

When you don't want goat does to kid on pasture or range they are moved into a maternity pen like that used for ewes. This is often dictated by poor weather, limited pasture, first kidding, or being bothered by other animals.

Sows

Sows are washed down with warm water and soap, concentrating on the genitals, flanks, underbelly, and teats—all of the areas that their piglets will come in contact with and where they could pick up parasite eggs. Then sows are moved from their gestation quarters to individual farrowing pens a couple of days before giving birth. These are generally located in a separate building and have been cleaned and disinfected. The farrowing house is maintained at 60–70° F [15.5–21° C] and is well lit and ventilated.

Signs Indicating Birth Will Take Place Soon

Beef and Dairy Cows

Starting several weeks before calving certain changes take place in the physical condition of pregnant cows (and more obviously in heifers) that should tip you off that they will be giving birth soon. The udder swells and the teats become distended. If the cow is normally a heavy milker and her udder is very full she may drip a little; if so, the milk will appear quite thick (since it is colostrum). The vulva swells as well, turns pinkish, and looks loose. The cow's abdomen appears much larger than normal. One to three days before calving the muscles on both sides of the tail, when looked at from the rear, will be observed to have sunk into the body, causing these areas to look softer and more relaxed than usually is the case.

Right before birth, in response to the first uterine contractions, the cow finds a secluded spot. She lies down and gets back to her feet over and over again, as if searching for a comfortable but unattainable position. Her behavior becomes increasingly nervous and she bellows and moans. The cow frequently turns her head back to peer at her rump and will occasionally kick at her abdomen. Sometimes a thick mucus is seen on the vulva. The cow arches her back and lifts her tail as if she were urinating.

Mares

Several weeks before foaling mares, like cows, fill up in the udder and their teats swell and distend. The muscles on both sides of the tail relax and become soft. Their vulvas swell, turn pinkish, and look loose and elastic.

Foaling is imminent when the mare, in response to the onset of uterine contractions, becomes nervous, lying down and getting to her feet repeatedly. She begins to sweat on the flanks about 4 hours before foaling, switches her tail back and forth, urinates often, and turns her head back to bite at her flanks.

Ewes

Ewe udders fill out well and the flesh in front of their hips sinks in during the last few weeks before lambing. As the first uterine contractions start, animals uneasily separate from the flock and look for a secluded spot. The vulva swells, turns pink, and looks loose. Ewes paw the ground, then lie down and get up frequently before lying down a final time to lamb. More lambings take place on the ground than standing up.

Goat Does

Does show easily recognizable signs of the approach of kidding. Their udders fill out and their teats distend very quickly. If this happens a week or more before kidding in heavy milkers you will probably have to strip out a little bit of milk each day to relieve the weight and discomfort of the heavy udder. Freeze this colostrum to feed to orphan lambs and to those whose mothers don't produce milk at kidding.

Several hours before kidding the flesh on both sides of the tail sinks into the body, the doe digs at her bedding, making a "nest," and she bleats a lot. Often does look backward, rest their heads on their backs, and talk to the kid(s) still in their uteruses. Just before birth their breathing speeds up and a colorless, mucus-like discharge is seen on the vulva. As the contractions come quicker does grunt and bleat at the same time. This is the best confirmation that kidding is now only minutes away.

Sows

In late pregnancy sows develop large abdomens. Four days before farrowing their vulvas swell, turn pinkish, and look loose. Their udders become full and functioning teats distend with milk 1-2 days before they give birth. The weight of the milk is often so great in large producers that they are unable to prevent letdown shortly before farrowing. Their teats are seen to drip and will occasionally release small streams. The skin of the udder becomes flushed and warm.

Up to a day before farrowing the sow becomes increasingly nervous and will nose about in her bedding, if she has any, arranging a "nest." She shifts from side to side when lying down, and stands and lies down repeatedly. About an hour before farrowing she becomes calmer, lies down, and doesn't move much until beginning her labor.

Normal Birth: Forelegs First

Cows, Mares, Ewes, Goat Does, and Sows

In the following description I have used a doe to describe the birth process, but the same sequence of events takes place in the cow, mare, ewe, and sow.

The first uterine contractions, which cause the goat to move about uneasily, change the position of the fetus. It moves from the bottom of the abdomen, where it has been lying flat, to an upright stance in front of the pelvis. The fetal waste fluids, held in a sac called the *first water bag,* are forced against the cervix with tremendous pressure by the uterine contractions. This causes the cervix to dilate (open wide). The first water bag and the fetus, enclosed by a fluid-filled membrane, are then forced through the cervix into the vagina.

The first water bag is pushed partially out of the vulva and bursts from the buildup of pressure. This is often called breaking water, and

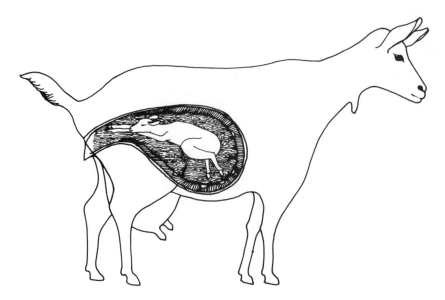

Figure 103.   The normal birth position (forelegs first).

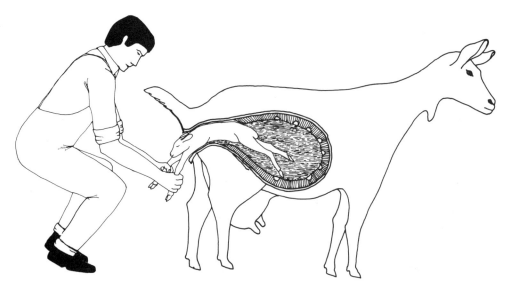

Figure 104.   In a front presentation, coordinate with the mother's pushes.

lubricates the birth canal. The muscular labor contractions are now applied to the fetus, forcing it forward toward the vulva. A portion of the
shiny white membrane emerges from the vulva and more and more of the
fluid is forced into it with the continuing contractions. At this point the
kid's legs can be seen through the membrane.

  The membrane (commonly called the *second water bag*) bursts and
bathes the vagina and vulva with its fluid. The doe pushes hard and forces
the kid's legs, head, and shoulders through the vulva. Then she often gets
to her feet and the kid slips out of the birth canal to the ground. The
normal position is for the kid to be born front legs first with its head resting in between them, almost as if it were diving out of the birth canal (see
Figures 103 and 104). As the front legs pass through the vulva the umbili-

cal cord breaks. This doesn't normally cause a problem because the goat quickly licks the pieces of membrane and the residue of the fluid from the kid's nostrils causing it to breathe.

If the kid breathes while still in the birth canal it will suffocate unless you quickly clean all membranes and fluid from its mouth and nostrils. Hold it upside down for a second to drain out this material while scooping it out with your fingers at the same time. Immediately start giving artificial respiration (if the kid hasn't yet breathed air) by holding your hand over the kid's mouth and gently blowing into its nostrils. Remove your hand and repeat this in 6–7 seconds. If there is still no respose find the flesh just to the side of the end of the rib cage and force your palm forward (in the direction of the head), and down several times in a row in this soft region. The normal involuntary muscular reaction when stimulated like this is to blow out and then to breathe in (as you no doubt realize if you have ever been hit in the stomach).

The doe licks its kid dry shortly after birth, which not only dries it but stimulates the doe to let down her milk. If the goat refuses to lick the kid dry or is too weak to do so, do it yourself with an old towel or burlap bag; but give the old girl a chance first. Then cut the umbilical cord an inch from the kid's belly with a sterilized knife or scissors, squeeze out a little blood and paint the cord with iodine.

The kid gets to its feet on rubbery legs and starts to search for a teat on its own or is nudged toward the udder by its mother. This often takes up to a few hours if the kid is left to its own devices, but if 30 minutes have gone by and the kid still hasn't nursed, give it a hand. The first milk, the colostrum, is rich in antibodies that the young animal needs to protect it from disease and has a laxative effect causing it to defecate, a very necessary body function after birth (see Figure 105).

Usually the afterbirth is expelled 2–6 hours after birth and the goat eats it. I don't think this should be discouraged (except in mares and sows) as the placenta and umbilical cord give her a quick shot of nutrients after a very great stress. Students of animal behavior claim this is a natural instinct in which the goat disposes of the evidence of the birth in order to hide the presence of its defenseless kid from predators.

Normal Birth: Hind Legs First

The emergence of the kid hindlegs first is also a normal birth position (see Figure 106). The one problem with a rear presentation (which you should immediately recognize when the hooves emerge upside down so that you can see the soles) is that the umbilical cord usually breaks when the kid is half way out of the birth canal. Since the normal reaction is to start breathing when the cord breaks, the kid may take its first breath while still inside the goat. This causes it to suck in pieces of membrane and fetal fluids instead of air, usually drowning it.

Since you certainly don't want to lose your kid crop through drowning, stick close by during kidding, and quickly size up whether it will be a front (forelegs first) or rear (hindlegs first) presentation. If it is the latter grasp each leg just under the hock and coordinate with the goat's pushes to firmly (but not roughly) pull the young animal downward toward its mother's hocks once it has emerged to the hips. Never pull straight out;

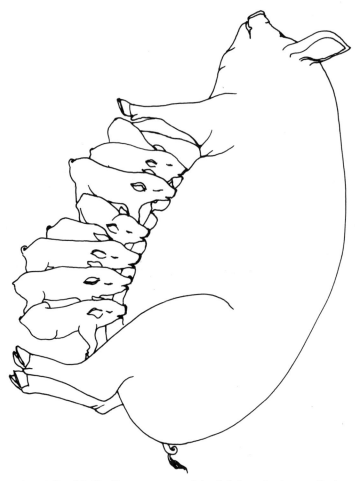

Figure 105.   After birth, the young need to drink colostrum, their mother's first milk.

the kid's shoulders won't be able to pass over the pelvis (see Figure 107). If the kid's shoulders are tight in the birth canal give it a quarter or half turn (so that its back is toward its mother's belly) and it should slip through more easily.

Once the kid has been delivered, hold it upside down and rapidly clean out its throat and nostrils, as previously described. Be sure when pulling the kid out that there is abundant straw underneath the goat to absorb the impact of its weight when it hits the ground. It is a heartbreaking experience, one you will never repeat, to assist in a successful rear presentation birth only to have the kid die on you when its head hits the concrete.

Normal Birth: Twins

Twins are quite normal in many sheep and goat breeds, and, of course, highly desirable. When selecting sheep and goats for breeding, twinning is very high on the list of characteristics you would like to build into your herd. Twinning is rare in horses and should be selected against

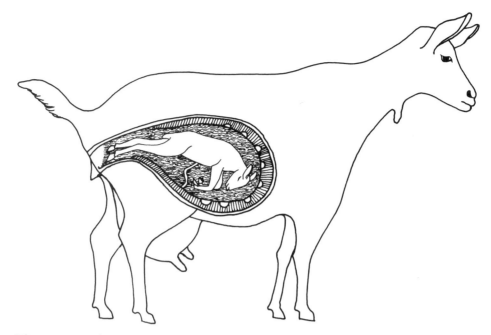

Figure 106.   The normal birth position (hind legs first).

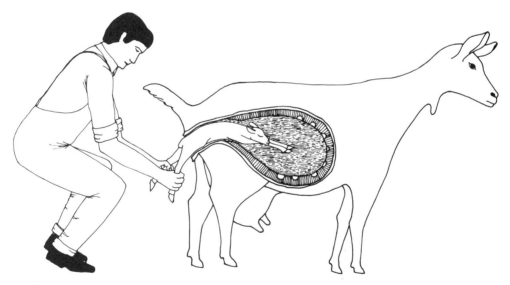

Figure 107.   In a rear presentation, coordinate with the mother's pushes.

as stillbirths are common in twin foals and half or less of them survive. In cattle, twinning is also discouraged because of the resultant sterility of a heifer born twin to a bull, as was discussed earlier the section on "Freemartins."

In twin births the first lamb or kid is almost always born in a front presentation (forelegs first), followed by a rear presentation in the second one (see Figure 108). You must assist in the rear presentation as you would in any other. Normally a doe or ewe licks the first kid or lamb dry after its birth and then leaves it to have the second one, but may return to nuzzle it between labor contractions.

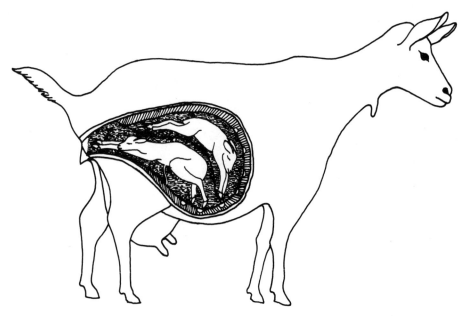

Figure 108.   The normal birth position for twins.

Problem Birth Positions

Animals need assistance during birth for many different problem positions. When the fetus is too large for the birth canal it is recommended that your veterinarian perform a caesarean operation. When the young die and swell in the uterus they must be cut into manageable sized pieces with an embryotomy knife by your veterinarian.

Assisting during a difficult birth is a skill that is only developed through practice with an experienced farmer or with your veterinarian. It takes common sense, a knowledge of the animal's anatomy, a level head, gentleness, and an understanding of your own limitations. Don't hesitate to call for help when you need it, and better yet, anticipate problem births by having the vet or an experienced friend standing by until you are secure on your own.

Anyone assisting with a difficult birth must follow a few basic rules.

1. Fingernails should by clipped short.
2. Remove rings, watches, and jewelry.
3. If the animal is longtailed, tie the tail to its neck to keep it out of the way.
4. Wash the animal's vulva with a mild soap and water before beginning.
5. If you use a cord disinfect it well.
6. Make sure there is enough light on the subject.
7. Scrub your hands and arms down well and disinfect them.
8. Use obstetrical lubricant or mineral oil to lubricate the birth canal, your hand, and your arm.
9. *Be gentle*—I can't emphasize this enough.

10. Once you have inserted your hand, identify the position of the fetus and think through the repositioning before you attempt it.
11. While repositioning the fetus never sever or break the umbilical cord or the fetus will drown.
12. Pull firmly (but not roughly) with the animal's labor exertions.
13. Always place an antibiotic bolus (large pill) in the female's uterus after removing a young animal.

Assistance should be given when animals appear in difficulty after laboring different lengths of time. Help will be needed when cows are in hard labor more than 2 hours; mares more than 1 hour; ewes more than 1½ hours; goat does for 30 minutes, and sows more than 2 hours.

Head Back

When the legs are forward for a frontal presentation and the head is turned back the head will catch on the pelvis. Put a cord noose around each leg and then gently push the kid back. Reach your hand in and move the head forward in between the legs. Pull on the cords in a downward motion to guide the legs and head towards the goat's hocks (see Figure 109).

One Front Leg Back

Attach a cord to the one leg that is in the normal position and another to the head (place the noose behind the ears and inside the mouth). Then gently push the fetus backward. Reach in with your hand and reposition the bent-back leg making sure the head is in between the legs (see Figure 110).

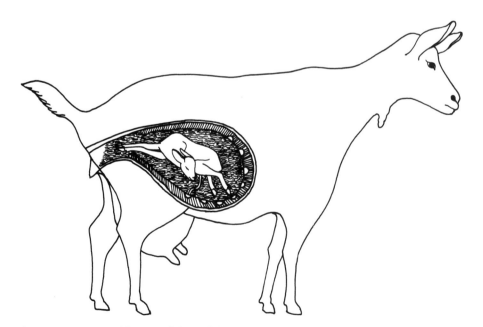

Figure 109.   A problem position with the head back.

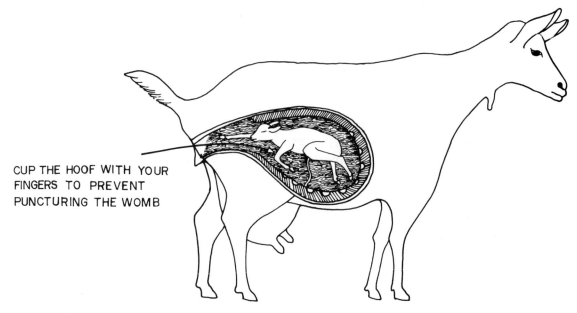

CUP THE HOOF WITH YOUR
FINGERS TO PREVENT
PUNCTURING THE WOMB

Figure 110.   A problem position with one front leg back.

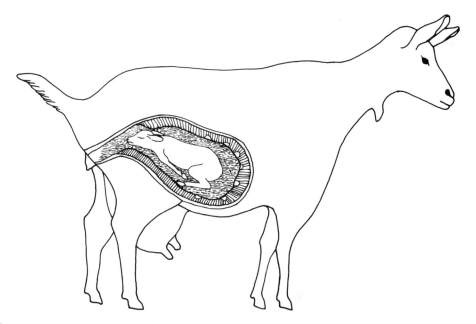

Figure 111.   A problem position with both front legs bent back.

Both Front Legs Back

Proceed as in the previous position by placing a noose around the head. Push the animal backward and reach in to reposition one leg followed by the other. Put a noose around each leg (see Figure 111). Sometimes it pays to raise the animal's rear, keeping the front of her body on

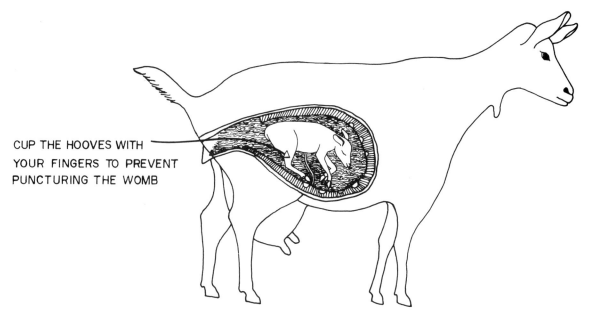

CUP THE HOOVES WITH
YOUR FINGERS TO PREVENT
PUNCTURING THE WOMB

Figure 112.   A problem position with both hind legs bent back.

the ground if there isn't enough space to get past the head with your hand or if you are afraid of puncturing the uterine wall when you bring a leg forward.

Rear Presentation with Both Hind Legs Back

Raise the animal's hindquarters, keeping her front on the ground. This will enable you to gently push the fetus backward in the uterus. With the added maneuvering space this gives, you'll be able to reach under the rump (of the fetus) and take hold of a leg. Bend it up at the hock so that the stifle, the part of the leg in front of and below the thigh, presses against the fetus's side. Then rotate the leg backward and into the proper birth position for a rear presentation. Be careful not to break the umbilical cord during this movement.

Repeat this with the other leg and put nooses around each one. Pull downward toward the mother's hocks (see Figure 112).

Two Front and Two Rear Legs with a Set of Twins

When one of a set of twins has its forelegs in the birth canal and the other has its hindlegs in the canal put a noose around the two forelegs (but make sure they belong to the same fetus). Then push both fetuses backward in the uterus, far enough to be able to maneuver the frontal presentation twin, with its head between its legs, into the birth canal. Deliver the frontal presentation twin first and then the rear presentation (see Figure 113).

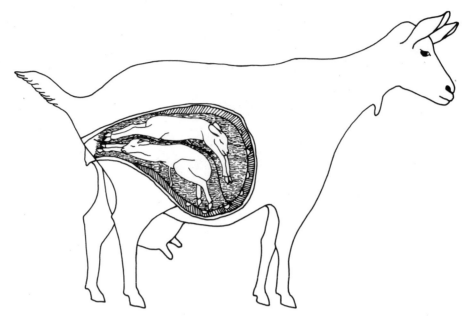

Figure 113.   A problem position in twins.

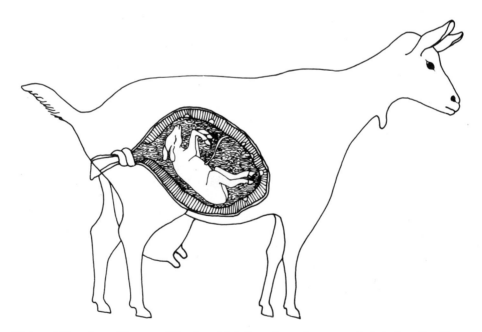

Figure 114.   A problem position in which the uterus becomes twisted on itself.

Torsion of the Uterus

Torsion is a real problem when it occurs. It happens when the uterus gets twisted on itself, usually in older ewes and goat does with twins, or even triplets. Late in pregnancy the weight of the multiple fetuses is heavy in the uterus and this causes it to flop over and turn on itself when the animal rolls over (see Figure 114). Now that you know what it is, I hope you never encounter it.

My only piece of advice on this is to quickly call your veterinarian. With any luck he or she won't have another emergency and will come running. Watch carefully what the vet does.

If the torsion involves the vagina they will reach their hand in to feel which way the twist goes, right or left. If the vagina is not involved and they can't tell which direction it goes in, they will do a rectal palpation to feel for the twist in the uterus. Once the direction has been determined the animal is laid down on the same side (on the right side for a twist to the right), with its fore- and hindlegs tied separately, and is then quickly rolled to the other side.

Another technique is to use a detorsion bar, which is a bar with a chain running its length that is looped over the fetus's legs if they can be reached. The animal is then turned while the fetus, and the uterus, are held in place by the bar.

These cases are very tricky and can sometimes only be resolved through a caesarean operation.

Follow-Up to Difficult Births

Weak young animals need help following birth. Make sure they get to their mother's udder quickly and that they get their fill of colostrum. If they have trouble finding a teat, put it in their mouth. Oftentimes they will suck but don't have the force to remove a plug of colostrum that is blocking the mother's nipple. So, quickly strip teats to open their nipples before the young nurse for the first time.

Keep your ears attuned for crying young after birth and for the next few days. It usually means they haven't nursed or, if they did, they might not have had enough milk. Sometimes they can't find the teat or are rejected by their mother. Often, newborn animals that are too weak to suck still have the strength to cry, albeit very weakly.

If young animals can't find a teat then help them do so. For all of the other problems bottle-feed them or transplant them to another lactating female (after feeding them some of the colostrum you've got sitting in the freezer for such situations). If they are too weak to nurse well strip out colostrum and bottle-feed them, but take care not to force milk into their lungs in your haste to get some into them. If they don't have a sucking reflex because of extreme weakness give them a dextrose injection (and possibly electrolytes) and feed again with the bottle in half an hour. If they are going to make it they usually start to suck.

Retained Placenta

Once females give birth they usually expel the membrane that has protected their offspring all through gestation within a few hours of the presentation. This membrane, called the *placenta* (and commonly, after the young are born, the afterbirth), is attached to the inner wall of the uterus by mushroomlike, spongy growths called *caruncles.*

If the afterbirth is not expelled within a reasonable time after birth (and at birth in the sow, since each piglet is normally born still encased in its own placenta) the animal is considered to have retained its placenta. All or part of the placenta is still attached to the uterine wall by the caruncles.

The afterbirth can be removed by hand by your veterinarian, but only if it sloughs off easily by peeling it from the uterine wall with a washed, disinfected, and lubricated hand. The peeling is done by slowly and gently moving your hand, from caruncle to caruncle, between the placenta and the uterine wall. If it doesn't come easily don't pull on it, even in the slightest. Should you rip the afterbirth from the uterine wall the animal will hemorrhage and possibly bleed to death: it usually becomes sterile. If the placenta is left in place and nothing is done to remove it the uterus will become infected and the animal may die. If it isn't possible for your veterinarian to remove the afterbirth by hand he or she can give the animal an injection which will cause the uterus to shed it. An antibiotic bolus is placed in the uterus to counter the possibility of infection and to dissolve pieces of the afterbirth.

The cervix must remain dilated for the afterbirth to pass through it and be expelled by the animal. For this reason it is important to observe births and watch for the passing of one afterbirth for each young animal born. The following guide should help you determine when your animals have retained their placentas:

WHEN PLACENTA SHOULD BE CONSIDERED RETAINED

Animal	A Placenta Is Retained If Not Expelled This Number of Hours After Birth
Cow	24
Mare	3
Ewe	12
Goat doe	12
Sow	12 (usually indicates that 1 or more piglets have yet to be born)

If a placenta has been retained beyond the number of hours mentioned in the table above, immediately call your veterinarian to begin treatment. There is no time to be lost since the cervix begins to close up tight within a few hours to days of these limits. When trapped in the uterus by a closed cervix the afterbirth decays and causes serious infection which can often become fatal.

Most commonly, a retained placenta is seen as a shiny, long, and stringy membrane hanging partially out of the vulva after birth. Less frequently the afterbirth is retained entirely inside the uterus, cervix, and birth canal so that no obvious signs are observed. Quickly get in the habit of counting placentas, and examine them to determine if any pieces have remained within the animal.

Prolapse of the Uterus

Prolapse, also called *eversion* (turning inside out), of the uterus is a very serious condition in which a female, after having given birth, continues to strain, as if still in labor, and forces her uterus out of her body by turning it inside out. You'll immediately know what has happened by the sight of the red, pouchlike uterus, the size of a basketball or shopping bag, covered with knoblike swellings (the caruncles) hanging from the vulva.

The animal immediately goes into shock and some die within a few minutes; others last a few days before dying if they aren't treated. Get on the phone to your vet and describe what has happened. Since they know it's an emergency in which a couple of minutes one way or the other are often crucial, they will be out the door as soon as you say "prolapse."

Meanwhile, get the animal into a private pen, if it isn't there already, but don't drive it hard or excite it since it's in shock. Have a helper wrap the uterus with a wet-down, warm towel and support its weight. While he or she does this you should build a slightly inclined ramp (a couple of feet higher at one end than the other) by propping up boards, a ladder, a sheet of plywood or any other sturdy, flat surface with hay bales. Back the animal up the inclined ramp so its rear is up in the air. This will take the weight and pressure off of the uterus.

By now your helper's arms are aching since the uterus is heavy. Lay a low bench or hay bale behind the animal's rear, cover it with a clean towel or sheet, and put the uterus on top of it. Keep the uterus wrapped with the wet towel. Bring a couple of buckets of warm water, some mild soap, and a bunch of clean towels into the pen.

Once the veterinarian arrives he or she gives the animal an anesthetic injection in the spine to reduce its straining and make the muscles relax. The uterus is carefully washed off and then placed back in its normal position by passing it through the vulva, vagina, and cervix with a washed, disinfected, and lubricated hand. This is a long, slow, painstaking process. Usually another anesthetic injection is given to stop the straining and to cause the uterus to shrink down after the reinsertion. The vulva is normally loosely sutured shut to prevent the forcing of the uterus through it once again. However, you should watch the animal carefully for several days and must call your veterinarian immediately if it starts straining because chances are good it will prolapse again if not treated promptly. No suture in the world will stop an animal from forcing its uterus through the vulva if it is straining hard.

Keep the animal's rear elevated in the pen on the temporary ramp you knocked together or build up one end of the pen with sand that is covered well with bedding. Make sure the animal is 1-2 feet higher in the rear than in the front.

Any animals that have prolapsed are prime candidates for culling since it is often a genetic problem. There is no sense in going through the same trouble and expense with them and their offspring year after year.

GLOSSARY

Abscess—a pus-filled spot in an animal's body, that may be swollen and inflamed, and is usually caused by a bacterial infection.

Acquired immunity—the resistance to a specific disease that develops after contracting it or by being vaccinated against it.

Active immunity—the resistance to a specific disease produced after having survived an attack of it.

Acute—occurs rapidly and lasts for a short period of time.

Afterbirth—the term by which the placenta is commonly known once the young animals have been born.

Anaerobic—only able to grow and multiply in the absence of air.

Anemia—a weakened state caused by three possible factors: 1) not enough red blood cells are made to replace the ones that have died; 2) the newly produced red blood cells do not contain enough hemoglobin; 3) the total amount of blood is less than normal.

Anestrus—when a female is not sexually receptive to a male of the species and does not show the typical signs of estrus associated with her species.

Anthrax—an infectious fever caused by a very powerful and fast-acting bacteria which frequently results in death.

Antibiotics—chemical compounds made by fungi, molds, and bacteria used to interfere with the growth or reproduction of attacking microorganisms or to kill them within the animal's body.

Antibody—a protein produced in response to an antigen (bacteria, toxin, enzyme, or other substance) that counteracts its effectiveness.

Antigen—a toxin, enzyme, bacteria, or chemical that causes the production of antibodies against a specific disease.

Antiseptic—a chemical compound that suppresses the activity and growth of microorganisms.

Antiserum—serum with antibodies in it that are specific to the disease being treated.

Antitoxins—proteins made by phagocytes that counteract the active properties of specific toxins, causing them to become ineffective.

Artificial insemination—the process in which the semen collected from the male of the species is passed into the uterus of the female in an artificial manner, usually with an AI straw.

Attenuated vaccines—vaccines made in the laboratory from living microorganisms that have been weakened.

Bacteria—one-celled microorganisms which may be beneficial, harmless, or disease-producing depending on the type.

Bacterin—a suspension of killed disease-causing bacteria placed in either a salt solution or oil that an animal is injected with to cause it to produce antibodies against a specific disease.

Biological products—substances produced in the laboratory or in animals' bodies used to give either immediate, temporary protection against attacking microorganisms, to cure an animal after infection, to cause a long-lasting immunity, or to detect and diagnose specific diseases.

Bang's Disease—a common name for Brucellosis in cattle.

Broad spectrum drugs—drugs that are effective against many different microorganisms.

Brucellosis—an infectious bacterial disease that can cause abortion and reproductive failure.

Canula—a small, round-tipped tube with one or more holes in its sides that is inserted into the teat to give an intramammary infusion.

Caruncles—the mushroom-like, spongy growths by which the placenta is attached to the inner wall of the uterus.

Castration—the operation in which the testicles of the male animal are surgically removed.

Chronic infection—an infection that lasts a long time or recurs frequently.

Circling Disease—a common name for Listeriosis.

Closed herd—a herd into which no outside animals are introduced for either breeding or replacement.

Colostrum—the first milk, rich in antibodies and protein, produced by a female animal for several days after giving birth.

Contagious Abortion—a common name for Brucellosis in cattle.

Crutching—to trim the wool from around a ewe's udder, flanks, and tail.

Cull—to remove an undesirable animal from a herd and dispose of it.

Disease carrier—an animal that carries an infection within its body but does not show any of the signs of infection.

Docking—to cut off the end of an animal's tail, usually done to lambs for health reasons and to facilitate the breeding of ewes when they become sexually mature.

Dormant—inactive.

Elastration—a process in which a small, thick rubber band is placed around a male's scrotum close to its groin cutting off the blood supply to it and the testicles; the testicles die, dry up, and fall off in a few weeks.

Emasculatome—an instrument used to crush a male's testicular cord and artery in order to cut off the blood supply to its testicles.

Endotoxins—poisons contained within harmful bacteria that are released when these die and break down.

Enteritis—inflammation of the intestines.

Enzymes—organic substances similar in composition to proteins that serve as catalysts by starting or speeding up certain chemical reactions.

Estrous cycle—the cyclical, hormone-influenced reproductive pattern of female animals.

External parasites—insects, fleas, lice, and ticks.

Facing—trimming the wool from a ewe's face.

Fibrinogen—a protein in blood plasma that is converted into a blood clot by the enzyme thrombin.

Final host—the animal within which an internal parasite completes its life cycle, attains maturity, and within which it may reproduce.

First water bag—a membrane, in the shape of a sac, that contains the fetal waste fluids.

Fistulas—passages or ducts formed in infected tissue leading to the surface of the skin, body cavities, or body organs.

Fistulous withers—a common name for a Brucella infection in horses in which the top of the back becomes inflamed.

Flatworm—a common name for the Platyhelminthes, a group of flat, soft, unsegmented worms that are often parasitic.

Foot and Mouth Disease—a severe and very infectious viral disease of cloven-hooved animals throughout the world whose typical symptoms are fever and blisters around the mouth and hooves.

Foot Scabies—a common name for Chorioptic Scabies, an infectious disease of the skin, the legs, feet, udder, and abdomen caused by tiny mites.

Freshening—to begin to give milk after giving birth.

Genetic inheritance—the collection of traits received by an animal from its parents and ancestors.

Gilt—a young sow that has not had its first litter yet.

Glanders—a contagious, usually fatal disease of horses, mules, donkeys, and burros in which the common symptoms are fever, inflammation, and lesions of the nasal tract, lungs, and skin.

Hemmorhage—loss of a large quantity of blood.

Hepatic—having to do with the liver.

Immune blood serum—blood serum containing antibodies against a specific disease produced by an actively immune animal that is injected into another animal to give it passive immunity against the same disease.

Immune bodies—antibodies.

Immunity—the power to resist a specific disease.

Inactivated vaccines—vaccines made from microorganisms that, although they have been killed by chemicals, stimulate a strong antibody response.

Individual immunity—the degree of immunity shown by a specific animal due to age and genetic inheritance.

Inflammation—a response to injury or infection in which the tissue becomes red, swollen, hot, and painful.

Intermediate host—the animal in which an internal parasite passes through the different stages of its larval development before reaching its final living place.

Internal parasites—forms of animal life that live inside animals and derive their nourishment from them for all or part of their existence.

Intradermal—between the layers of the skin.

Intramammary—into the teat.

Intramuscular—into a muscle.

Intraperitoneal—into the abdominal cavity.

Intrarumen—into the rumen.

Intravenous—into a vein.

Kindling—giving birth in rabbits.

Leptospirosis—a contagious bacterial disease of horses, cattle, pigs, sheep, goats, and man that produces many symptoms ranging from fever and anemia to abortion and death.

Listeriosis—a bacterial disease in many animal varieties and man that may cause abortion or central nervous system injuries.

Live vaccines—vaccines made in the laboratory from living microorganisms that have been weakened.

Lockjaw—a common name for Tetanus.

Mange—a disease of the tissue under the outer surface of the skin caused by mites.

Mastitis—an inflammation of the mammary gland of a female animal that may be caused by many kinds of bacteria and yeasts.

Monoestrus—having one estrus cycle each year.

Moon Blindness—an intermittent disease of the eyes in horses which is suspected of being caused by Leptospira bacteria.

Natural species immunity—the natural immunity that animals have against a specific disease because it does not affect their species.

Newcastle Disease—an acute viral infection in fowl whose common symptoms are respiratory problems, pneumonia, central nervous system damage, and death in chicks.

Nitrofurans—man-made chemicals made from peanut shells, oat hulls, corn cobs, and beet pulp that are used to kill many kinds of bacteria.

Obstetrical sleeve—a long plastic glove used to palpate with.

Orchitis—when one or both of the testicles are larger than normal.

Palpation—to explore by feeling, usually done to check for pregnancy.

Passive immunity—the immunity produced in an animal by injecting it with the immune blood serum taken from another animal.

Pasteurellosis—an infectious bacterial disease whose symptoms are pneumonia, inflammation of the lungs, or septicemia.

Pathogenic—disease causing.

Peracute—very severe, occurs extremely rapidly, and lasts for a short period of time.

Periodic Ophthalmia—an intermittent disease of the eyes in horses, more commonly called Moon Blindness, which is suspected of being caused by Leptospira bacteria.

Peritoneum—thin, watery membrane that lines the abdominal cavity.

Peritonitis—inflammation of the peritoneum.

Phagocytes—white blood cells that destroy microorganisms, other cells, and any foreign matter in the blood and body tissues.

Placenta—the membrane attached to the uterine wall of the pregnant female and to the developing embryo by the umbilical cord, within which the fetus develops.

Plasma—the fluid remaining when red and white blood cells are removed from the blood.

Poll Evil—a Brucella infection in horses in which the top of the head becomes inflamed.

Polyestrous—having more than one estrous cycle a year.

Prolapse—when a female, after having given birth, continues to strain, as if still in labor, forces her uterus out of her body, turning it inside out.

Protozoa—one-celled animals that mainly live in water, some of which are parasitic.

Quarantine—to isolate animals suspected of or suffering from contagious diseases from their herdmates.

Rabies—an infectious viral disease that attacks the central nervous system and whose symptoms are frothing at the mouth, an inability to swallow liquids, rage, convulsions, and choking.

Redwater—a common name for Leptospirosis in calves.

Relapse—the recurrence of an illness.

Renal—having to do with the kidneys.

Roundworm—a variety of Nematode worm that lives as a parasite in animals' intestines.

Scab—a disease of the tissue under the outer surface of the skin caused by mites; also called Mange.

Scabies—a contagious disease of the surface of the skin caused by mites.

Schistosomiasis—a disease caused by thin, 1⅕″ long parasitic flukes that live in the blood vessels.

Seasonal breeders—animals that always come into heat once a year, and hence are monoestrus, at the same time unless under great stress.

Secondary bacterial invaders—bacteria present in an animal's body that attack it once the animal's natural defenses have been lowered by a previous viral infection.

Selective drug—a drug used to counteract a particular harmful microorganism; also called a specific drug.

Septicemia—blood poisoning.

Second water bag—the fluid-filled membrane that encloses the fetus and that bursts, lubricating the vagina and vulva before the young animal is expelled from its mother's body during birth.

Serum—the clear to yellowish liquid that separates from a blood clot when it begins to harden and shrink; it is made by removing the red and white blood cells and fibrinogen from the blood.

Silent heat—when a female shows no physical signs of estrus but actually is in heat.

Specific drugs—another term for selective drugs.

Split estrous—when a female animal comes into heat for a few days and lets the male mount her, then refuses to breed for a short period and finally, once again is receptive.

Standing heat—the period when a female will let the male mount her.

Sterile—a surface or environment without any living microorganisms on or in it.

Stomatitis—inflammation of the mouth.

Subclinical—without apparent symptoms.

Subcutaneous—directly below the skin and above the flesh.

Sulfa drugs—another term for sulfonamide drugs.

Sulfonamides—man-made drugs effective against a wide range of harmful bacteria.

Systemic treatment—treating the whole body; i.e., through the bloodstream.

Tetanus—a nervous system disease caused by a toxin produced by *Clostridium tetani* bacteria in most animals when they receive deep puncture wounds or become infected during castrations, dockings, or during birth via the umbilical cord.

Toxins—poisons produced by pathogenic microorganisms.

Toxoids—toxins that have been altered by chemicals or heat so they are no longer poisonous but still retain their antigenic properties.

Trichomoniasis—a disease in cattle, whose typical symptoms are infertility and abortion, caused by whiplike, parasitic protozoa.

Trocar—a pointed instrument used to make a hole in the animal's stomach in the case of bloat.

Tuberculosis—a highly infectious disease produced by the tubercle bacillus causing hard swellings in different tissues depending on the part of the body that is affected.

Vaccine—a preparation of a living, but weakened or diluted, virus that is injected into an animal's body to intentionally infect it with a mild form of disease in order to stimulate the production of antibodies.

Vaccination—the injection of a vaccine into an animal's body.

Virus—a microscopic living organism considered to be a complex protein that lives and reproduces within living cells.

Wryneck—the central nervous system form of Listeriosis in fowl in which the neck becomes twisted and the head is held to one side as a result of frequent contractions of the neck muscles.

INDEX